Social Work Practice in Pediatric Palliative and End-of-Life Care

As an essential and emerging practice, pediatric palliative care seeks to prevent and relieve suffering for children with life-threatening conditions. Palliative care teams are composed of providers of various disciplines, including social workers and their families, who collaborate to address the medical, social-emotional, and spiritual needs of the child, and their families. Social workers are especially accustomed to interdisciplinary care and may counsel, provide resources, facilitate communication, and promote person- and family-centered practices that are the basis of effective pediatric palliative care. This book presents practice strategies, experiential knowledge, and research related to practicing in collaborative teams, ICU settings, and hospice. It also presents research that is informed by the perceptions and perspectives of bereaved parents, parents who have suffered a stillbirth, and parent caregivers of children with life-limiting illness. This book highlights the unique role social workers play, within care teams and in relationships with children who have life-limiting illness, and their families.

This book was originally published as a special issue of the *Journal of Social Work in End-of-Life & Palliative Care*.

Barbara L. Jones, PhD, is Associate Professor, Assistant Dean for Health Affairs, and Co-Director of the Institute for Grief, Loss, and Family Survival in the School of Social Work at The University of Texas at Austin, USA. Her current research focuses on issues of pediatric palliative care, grief and loss, adolescent and young adult cancer survivorship, and the role of social work in health care.

W0234965

Social Work Practice in Pediatric Palliative and End-of-Life Care

Challenges and Opportunities

Edited by

Barbara L. Jones

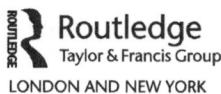
Routledge
Taylor & Francis Group

LONDON AND NEW YORK

First published in paperback 2024

First published 2015
by Routledge
4 Park Square, Milton Park, Abingdon, Oxon, OX14 4RN

and by Routledge
605 Third Avenue, New York, NY 10158

Routledge is an imprint of the Taylor & Francis Group, an informa business

Publisher's Note
The publisher has gone to great lengths to ensure the quality of this reprint but points out that some imperfections in the original copies may be apparent.

Disclaimer
Every effort has been made to contact copyright holders for their permission to reprint material in this book. The publishers would be grateful to hear from any copyright holder who is not here acknowledged and will undertake to rectify any errors or omissions in future editions of this book.

British Library Cataloguing in Publication Data
A catalogue record for this book is available from the British Library

ISBN: 978-1-138-77876-4 (hbk)
ISBN: 978-1-03-293086-2 (pbk)
ISBN: 978-1-315-77165-6 (ebk)

DOI: 10.4324/9781315771656

Typeset in Garamond
by Taylor & Francis Books

Contents

Citation Information

The chapters in this book were originally published in the *Journal of Social Work in End-of-Life & Palliative Care*, volume 8, issue 4 (December 2012). When citing this material, please use the original page numbering for each article, as follows:

Chapter 6
"I'll Never Forget Those Cold Words as Long as I Live": Parent Perceptions of Death Notification for Stillbirth
Suzanne Pullen, Mindi Ann Golden, and Joanne Cacciatore
Journal of Social Work in End-of-Life & Palliative Care, volume 8, issue 4 (December 2012) pp. 339–355

Chapter 7
Informing Social Work Practice Through Research With Parent Caregivers of a Child With a Life-Limiting Illness
Susan Cadell, Kimberly Kennedy, and David Hemsworth
Journal of Social Work in End-of-Life & Palliative Care, volume 8, issue 4 (December 2012) pp. 356–381

Please direct any queries you may have about the citations to
clsuk.permissions@cengage.com

Notes on Contributors

Eugene Aisenberg, School of Social Work, University of Washington, Seattle, Washington, USA

Joanne Cacciatore, School of Social Work, Arizona State University, Phoenix, Arizona, USA

Susan Cadell, School of Social Work, Renison University College, University of Waterloo, Waterloo, Ontario, Canada

J. Randall Curtis, Department of Medicine, Division of Pulmonary and Critical Care Medicine, School of Medicine, University of Washington, Seattle, Washington, USA

Ardith Doorenbos, Department of Biobehavioral Nursing & Health Systems, School of Nursing, University of Washington, Seattle, Washington, USA

Katherine Gilmore, Department of Symptom Research, The University of Texas MD Anderson Cancer Center, Houston, Texas, USA

Mindi Ann Golden, Communication Studies, San Francisco State University, San Francisco, California, USA

Ross Hays, Center for Child Health, Behavior and Development, Seattle Children's Research Institute, and Department of Rehabilitative Medicine, School of Medicine, University of Washington, Seattle, Washington, USA

David Hemsworth, Faculty of Applied & Professional Studies, School of Business & Economics, Nipissing University, North Bay, Ontario, Canada

Barbara L. Jones, School of Social Work, The University of Texas at Austin, USA

Kimberly Kennedy, Faculty of Social Work, Wilfrid Laurier University, Kitchener, Ontario, Canada

Taryn Lindhorst, School of Social Work, University of Washington, Seattle, Washington, USA

Riza Mauricio, Division of Pediatrics, The University of Texas MD Anderson Cancer Center Children's Cancer Hospital, Houston, Texas, USA

Shirley Morrison, Department of Nursing, Texas Women's University Houston Center, Houston, Texas, USA

Noam Ostrander, MSW Program, DePaul University, Chicago, Illinois, USA

Guadalupe R. Palos, Office of Cancer Survivorship, The University of Texas MD Anderson Cancer Center, Houston, Texas, USA

Suzanne Pullen, Hugh Downs School of Human Communication, Arizona State University, Tempe, Arizona, USA

Stacy S. Remke, School of Social Work, University of Minnesota, St. Paul, Minnesota, USA

Rhonda Robert, Division of Pediatrics, The University of Texas MD Anderson Cancer Center Children's Cancer Hospital, Houston, Texas, USA

Martha M. Schermer, School of Social Work, University of Minnesota, St. Paul, Minnesota, USA

Helene Starks, Department of Bioethics and Humanities, School of Medicine, University of Washington, Seattle, Washington, USA

Martha Vargas, MSW Program, DePaul University, Chicago, Illinois, USA

Donna S. Zhukovsky, Division of Pediatrics, The University of Texas MD Anderson Cancer Center Children's Cancer Hospital, Houston, Texas, USA, and Department of Palliative Care and Rehabilitation Medicine, The University of Texas MD Anderson Cancer Center, Houston, Texas, USA

INTRODUCTION

I am delighted to be Guest Editor for this special issue of the *Journal of Social Work in End-of-Life and Palliative Care*. This issue is a timely discussion of the state of pediatric palliative care social work. Pediatric palliative care has grown considerably in the past decade since the Institute of Medicine report *When Children Die* (2002) that stated that care for children was not "compassionate, consistent, nor competent." Since that report, there has been a proliferation of pediatric palliative care programs in children's hospitals throughout the country. Pediatric palliative medicine is now recognized as a subspecialty certification from the American Board of Medical Specialties and a certification from the Joint Commission for hospital palliative care programs. Educational programs, multidisciplinary research, and evidence-informed practice in this highly specialized field have also grown in response. Social workers have been integral as part of pediatric palliative care teams and leaders in advancing practice, research, and education. I hope you will be inspired by the articles presented in this issue.

The issue opens with a reflective piece by Vargas and Ostrander that details the lead author's experience learning to be a social worker in pediatric hospice care. Her initial reluctance but eventual gratitude for the work remind us all about why we began and why we continue to practice in palliative care.

Next is an invited article by Remke and Schermer on interprofessional team collaboration in pediatric palliative care. Given the increasing focus on transdisciplinary teamwork and interprofessional education in health care and especially in palliative care, Remke and Schermer offer a review of the literature and illustrative case examples for consideration. They highlight the importance of careful attention to team dynamics and management with the patient and family at the center of decision making and care planning. The skills of social work are essential in creating and communicating in interprofessional teams.

This special issue also offers four peer-reviewed articles examining many aspects of palliative care for children and their families. These articles all demonstrate the growing research in pediatric palliative care that is aimed at improving practice every day. First, Doorenbos and colleagues discuss the unique challenges of providing family-centered palliative care in Pediatric Intensive Care Units (PICU) and offer empirically-based recommendations for improving care. In the fast-paced environment of the PICU, practitioners

1

face many competing demands including the intensity of the care, the urgent and important family needs for information, support and communication, and the multiple and ever changing goals of care. Social workers in PICUs play a key role in helping families stay informed, updated, involved, and supported. The authors offer a review of empirically based approaches to family-centered palliative care in the PICU and highlight the importance of building partnerships with families using these principles.

The next three articles provide evidence-informed insight into parental perspectives about care for children facing life-limiting conditions. First, Robert and colleagues report on their study of bereaved parents' perspectives of pediatric palliative care in pediatric oncology. Their study has a specific focus on parental experiences, expectations, and recommendations for improving care. The interdisciplinary team conducted three focus groups with a total of 14 parents at a southwestern NCI-designated cancer center. Families' responses focused on the themes of standards of care, emotional care, communication, and social support. Robert and colleagues suggest recommendations for clinical social workers to incorporate these findings into care delivery. Additionally, they promote the increased teaching of pediatric palliative care in masters and post-master's training programs that include the voices of parents.

Pullen and colleagues report on a qualitative study of parental positive and negative experiences with health care providers following a stillbirth. In this retrospective study, the authors examined the open-ended survey responses of parents who had expressed a strong opinion about how they received notification of their baby's death. Using a constant comparative approach, Pullen and colleagues found that the opposing groups received very different levels of support for emotions, continuity of care, and delivery of information. The authors' clinical suggestions based on these data suggest that providers should focus on providing clear language, empathy, acknowledgment of parent experience, and coordinated care. Listening to the voices of parents who have had very good and really poor experiences will guide us as we improve our systems of care.

Finally, Cadell and colleagues present findings from their multinational, mixed-methods study of posttraumatic growth of parents caring for a child with a life-limiting illness (LLI). In it, they report on the questionnaire and interview responses of 273 parent caregivers of children in Canada and the United States. Focusing on the potential for growth, healing, and resilience in families fits into the strengths-based approach of clinical social work. The authors identified two main themes in their findings: the high financial stress of parental caregivers of children with LLI and the posttraumatic growth of these caregivers. Specifically, these parent caregivers reported that they faced enormous financial challenges; experienced growth at the same time as distress; built connections with other families; became advocates for their children; and developed strategies for self-care. Cadell and colleagues encourage social workers in pediatric palliative care to enhance the identified strategies that may lead other parents to experience growth while simultaneously experiencing the adversity of facing their child's LLI.

This special edition offers a unique focus on pediatric palliative care social work. The voices of parents are an essential component of much of the current research being conducted by social workers. Parents teach us that while there has been considerable improvement in care, there is still room for improvement in care coordination, communication, empathy, and strategies that recognize and enhance familial growth. The next steps in research should include more voices of extended family members such as grandparents, aunts, and the perspectives of the children themselves. And despite an increase in educational offerings in the past 10 years, each of these articles reflected that there is still a need for more specialized training in graduate schools of social work and post-master's education. While we are always learning from the children and families we serve, we can better prepare social workers before they enter the practice of pediatric palliative care. Taken together, these articles highlight the incredible strength of children and families and the deep commitment of social workers providing pediatric palliative care. I look forward to the next decade of reducing the need for palliative care for children and improving care for those who do need it.

Barbara L. Jones

Learning to Be: Reflections of a Social Work Student on a Pediatric Hospice Internship

MARTHA VARGAS and NOAM OSTRANDER

MSW Program, DePaul University, Chicago, Illinois, USA

INTRODUCTION

End-of-life and hospice care challenges the emotional strength of all social workers who provide care to dying individuals and their family members. These challenges may be amplified for social work interns who are not only new to the field of social work, but also new to the field of hospice and palliative care. Many of these students are enrolled in social work programs that lack adequate course offerings in the subject of death and dying (Huff, Weisenfluh, Murphy, & Black, 2006). This lack of formalized instruction can often require additional support and supervision from field instructors and individual faculty members. As a result, there are key areas where social work students feel underprepared—such as discussing the transition from curative care to palliative care, advocating around symptom management and pain control, and providing education about the illness's likely progression (Jones, 2005).

In many ways, this information about the preparation gaps for social work students mirrored my own experiences in my hospice internship. I can recall that when I initially interviewed for my internship at a hospice agency, one of the most important things to me was that I did not want to work with children. Being a mother of two children myself, I felt that working with sick children and their families was something that would be much too difficult for me. Although I understood that as a social work intern and later as a professional social worker I would face difficult situations, working with children was not something that I wanted to challenge myself to do. I had

The authors would like to thank Zayda Stewart for her wisdom, support, and encouragement throughout the hospice internship.

worked at a school for several years prior and although it was something I enjoyed I had a very hard time accepting and understanding the way that children are often treated. In this situation where I would be working with children who were sick and also dying, I felt that I would definitely not be able to handle these situations. I am now glad that my field instructor felt differently and had confidence that I could serve families with sick and dying children. Because of that confidence, I learned three valuable lessons about working with pediatric patients and their families.

LESSON 1: "SOMETIMES YOU HAVE TO JUST BE WITH THE FAMILY"

I was an intern at the hospice agency for approximately one month and was assigned several patients. As time went on, I was seeing a lot more children, especially Spanish-speaking families because I am bilingual. There were many lessons learned with each family but I think there were some that were more salient than others. My first pediatric patient was a young 16-year-old girl who was diagnosed with Rett Syndrome, a genetic disorder that affects mainly girls. I remember thinking to myself that I was going to go on one visit just to show my instructor that I had attempted to do this, but this was not something that I would be doing long term. I was very wrong. I followed this patient my entire internship and ended up having to transition the case back to my field instructor. I really enjoyed meeting with this family and learning from them.

My initial visits with the family were mainly with the patient's mom, but as time went on I met her siblings and her stepfather. My visits were very consistent; we met every other week, usually on Friday mornings. Many of our visits were to provide support. This would be when I learned my first lesson. Initially I thought I was going there to make a huge change or to do something important. However, my field instructor would often say, "Sometimes you have to just *be* with the family." I had no idea what this meant and I figured I would have some task to do when going to visit the families. I learned quickly what it meant to just be. There was not much that I could do to change the situation the families were in and obviously there was nothing that I could do to change their child's condition. What I could do was to be a supportive listener. Oftentimes I would not say much, I would mainly listen. I saw with many families that when children became ill, the parents often became separated from their extended family and friends due to the time spent caring for their child. I also observed that it can become difficult for family members to support another family member whose child is dying. As a hospice social worker, this is often the role we have to fill. We need to be that individual to listen and provide support. I found that some-times during my visits with families, the moms simply enjoyed talking about their day and their child. I did not think I was performing a monumental task, or even doing anything, oftentimes I would just be.

LESSON 2: TO THE CHILD'S PARENTS THEY ARE JUST THEIR CHILD WHOM THEY LOVE DEEPLY

The second child I was assigned was a 4-month-old baby girl who was born with a genetic disorder. Nothing could have prepared me for the emotions that went though me when I met this family. I was so sad for them. I had two healthy children myself, and I thought it was so unfair that such a nice young couple could not have the same healthy children I enjoyed. They were a young couple: the mom was 21 years old and the dad was 24 years old. This was their first baby and the first grandchild for the family. I remember that when I sat with them, it took everything in me not to cry with the mom as she told me about her baby and how much she loved her.

It was Christmas time and they were looking forward to having her home for the holidays, which they had accomplished. I was not sure what to expect when I saw her, but she looked like every other baby I had seen. This is also how her parents saw her: as their normal baby. This would be the second lesson that I learned from working with pediatric hospice patients. To the child's parents they are just their child whom they love deeply. Although parents know that their children are sick and oftentimes dying, they see their children as just being their children. I saw that the families learned to embrace every moment they have with their child. One perfect example of this was with the mom of this baby. I called her to schedule a visit and she informed me that she would not be able to meet because she was going to an appointment at WIC and she had to take the baby with her. I was glad that I called when I did because the nurse had recommended not taking the baby out in the cold and especially not where there were many other people due to the risk of infection. The mom responded to me that she thought all babies had to go and they would not give her coupons if she did not take the baby. She was not thinking that her baby was sick, all she was thinking was that all babies went to the first appointment. I was able to get a waiver for her so she did not need to bring her baby to the WIC office. This was the first time that I really understood that some parents did not see their children the way others did: not as a sick child but rather as their baby.

LESSON 3: FAMILIES HAVE AN INCREDIBLE AMOUNT OF STRENGTH

I think that one of the most difficult cases for me was when I was assigned to a 16-year-old girl who had a brain tumor and had been receiving treatment for some time. After having visited many patients, I was not sure what to expect when meeting the family and I knew how difficult cancer could be not only for adults but also for children. My grandmother had died from complications due to cancer and it was difficult for me to see her go through treatments. When I first met with the patient and her mother it reminded me of my grandmother's experience with cancer. The young girl had lost her hair from the treatment and she had some swelling, the same way my grandmother did. I think that this is what made this situation so much more difficult; I was already dealing with my own emotions in regards to cancer and then there was so much loss for this family. The patient's mom had recently experienced the death of her husband and shortly after, her daughter was diagnosed with a brain tumor. While this was a very difficult situation—the family had experienced such a huge loss and now they were preparing for another—it was also a significant learning experience. The strength and resiliency of this mother was amazing. I oftentimes would wonder if I would be able to handle so much loss in my own life.

I was able to learn a lot about this mother and really admired her for being able to hold everything together. Throughout her husband's illness, she had to work because he was no longer able to do so due to his leukemia. Thus, she had to become the provider for the family. When her daughter became ill, the mom now had to stop working to care for her daughter. She was an undocumented immigrant and really struggled. However, she managed to maintain her home, her family, and her sanity. She had family members who were able to move in with her to help her keep her home and assist with household chores. She would oftentimes say that she was able to handle everything because she had to and what she had to endure was nothing compared to what her daughter was going through.

One thing that I always found very difficult was that she always felt that her daughter was doing better and that she could get better. The hopeful part of me wanted that to be true but when I heard medical reports or would ask questions about her illness, I knew that this was not the case. This mom was able to get her daughter into rehabilitation to help with her walking but it did not improve much. In addition, the young girl had lost the ability to communicate due to the treatments and the illness. This mom was able to get a second opinion on her daughter's treatment and services that she felt her daughter needed, despite doctors saying there was nothing to improve her condition. This was a mother who did not speak English fluently but she was able to get what she needed if it meant her daughter would get better. She had strength not only to deal with the emotions associated with her daughter's illness but also to navigate a medical system that can oftentimes be difficult to maneuver for someone who speaks English and has resources. This would be another lesson that I learned while working in hospice and palliative care: families—especially parents—have an incredible amount of strength to cope with what they are enduring. As pediatric hospice social workers, we have to prop up that strength to provide support and help families through the death of a child.

FINAL REFLECTIONS

With these three families in particular I learned lessons that would really help me when working with all the pediatric patients I served at the agency and will serve in the future. Perhaps the most important lesson was how to deal with my own emotions and not feel guilty for having healthy children at home. These three families had not done anything to make their children sick and were very nice people who had the same hopes for their children that I do for mine, but their hopes changed. It was very important for me to be able to have supervision and be able to discuss my feelings about the cases with my field instructor. It was also important for me to be able to understand that it was appropriate for me to be sad and also grieve some of the losses of the children especially when I had spent so much time with the children and the families.

Working with children was something that I never thought I would want to do, especially children who were sick and dying. I have found that these experiences have made me a better social worker, and truly what you take away from the experience of working with these families is so much more than I could ever give to them. I cannot recall where it was that I heard this piece of wisdom, but one way of looking at this work is that when babies are born there are so many people present to greet them into this world. However, there are often not that many people willing to be there to say goodbye as they leave this world. When we work in hospice and palliative care we have that honor.

REFERENCES

Huff, M., Weisenfluh, S., Murphy, M., & Black, P. (2006). End-of-life care and social work education: What do students need to know? *Journal of Gerontological Social Work, 48*(1–2), 219–231.

Jones, B. (2005.) Pediatric palliative and end-of-life care: The role of social work in pediatric oncology. *Journal of Social Work in End-of-Life & Palliative Care, 1*(4), 35–62.

Team Collaboration in Pediatric Palliative Care

STACY S. REMKE

School of Social Work, University of Minnesota, St. Paul, Minnesota, USA

MARTHA M. SCHERMER

Children's Hospitals and Clinics of Minnesota, St. Paul, Minnesota, USA

This article explores themes related to team development in pediatric palliative care. A review of the literature, observations from the field, and an analysis of dynamics from the point of view of the social work knowledge base are included. Recommendations for team development and sustainability are shared.

INTRODUCTION

The specialty field of pediatric palliative care (PPC) has been growing rapidly in recent years, in parallel with the specialty practice of hospice and palliative medicine. Different models of care have been evolving. The interdisciplinary model of care that began as an outgrowth of hospice care has become the gold standard and palliative care is increasingly seen as a best practice for care in pediatrics, allowing palliative interventions to be offered along with curative or life-prolonging measures. More importantly, this care may extend over years. Collaboration between professionals of different disciplines represented on the PPC specialty care team is seen as a hallmark of pediatric palliative care, yet there is little training or guidance available to teams on how they might become effective together.

A review of the literature offers insight as to how challenges to team-work might arise and also offers guidance as to how to develop and sustain effective team functioning. The "care and feeding" of the team is an essential program activity that requires planning, facilitation, and resources.

LITERATURE REVIEW

A review of the literature reflects growing interest in the issues involved with developing and sustaining effective team functioning in palliative care. The process of the evolution of palliative care teams as an outgrowth of concepts from hospice care are described (Youngwerth & Twaddle, 2011). The presence of interdisciplinary teams in palliative care is correlated with positive outcomes (Youngwerth & Twaddle, 2011; O'Connor & Fisher, 2011; Blacker & Deveau, 2010). There is little research to date on how teams communicate or optimally function (O'Connor & Fisher, 2011). Teams have been variously described as interdisciplinary, multidisciplinary, and more recently, interprofessional (Blacker & Deveau, 2010). The complexity of teamwork in the context of medical culture is evident, and barriers to effective teamwork include the traditional medical model, hierarchy, the lack of training in collaborative practice, and competing values (Abramson & Mizrahi, 2003). Patient and family priorities for a multidisciplinary approach to their complex needs are also found in the literature (Abramson & Mizrahi, 2003). In cases of serious and life-threatening illness, patient and family needs tend to be too complex for any single discipline to address (Abramson & Mizrahi, 2003). Professionals from different disciplines often do not understand each other's roles and skills (Abramson & Mizrahi, 2003). Collaborative models of care that empower patients and families to participate actively in their care are the preferred methods of collaboration in pediatrics (Zimmerman & Dabelko, 2007; Feudtner, 2007). Team collaboration in the context of family-centered care models for care are associated with positive outcomes including safer care, better communication, and improved compliance with treatment (Zimmerman & Dabelko, 2007; http://teamstepps.ahrq.gov). It has also been identified that social workers possess skills and knowledge that can facilitate effective teamwork (Zimmerman & Dabelko, 2007; Jones, 2005).

Pediatric palliative care team dynamics have been evolving in a context of rapid growth and change in the hospice and palliative care movement. What was once care delivered through home-based services, or perhaps through an enlightened single practitioner is now increasingly being delivered through hospital-based consultation programs, often in partnership with community-based home, palliative, or hospice care providers. Educational programs have been developed to teach program development strategies (http://www.capc.org) and also clinical skills (e.g.: ELNEC-Pediatrics, NHPCO PPC Curriculum, ExCEL in social work). However, while interdisciplinary team care is seen as a core concept in palliative care, little training exists regarding how to participate in, or manage interdisciplinary team dynamics (Youngwerth & Twaddle, 2011). Also, little guidance is available as to how teams actually collaborate to make a difference in care. In fact, while studies demonstrate that interdisciplinary team care is tied to improved outcomes (Youngwerth & Twaddle, 2011; O'Connor & Fisher, 2011; Blacker & Deveau, 2010), there is little research to-date on how professionals communicate with each other about patients (O'Connor & Fisher, 2011), or how they work together. New models of "interprofessional collaboration" (IPC) are emerging that may offer guidance for team development (Blacker & Deveau, 2010). While not likely to rely on a single factor, the quality of team functioning seems to depend upon communication, interpersonal relations, team composition and structure, as well as organizational factors that impact the team (Youngwerth & Twaddle, 2011).

The traditional medical model is based upon a physician leader with allied professionals playing a supporting role (O'Connor & Fisher, 2011). Youngwerth and Twaddle (2011) described the evolving field of palliative care as a meeting of the cultures of the medical model and the hospice model. In hospice teams a "flatter" hierarchy of professional roles than seen in the traditional medical model can contribute to more effective access to knowledge from all the professionals on the team. This model of interprofessional collaboration (IPC) is based upon a shared appreciation of, and understanding of the roles and skills that each member brings to the team (Blacker & Deveau, 2010). The IPC model operates differently from traditional medical services in a hospital setting, with the contributions of each discipline equally valued and endorsed. Emerging teams can discuss and educate each other about their role's perspective, skill sets, and knowledge base. As teams grow in size, add and lose members, care for increasing volumes of patients, and manage the clinical intensity and complexity of illness that PPC often addresses, pressures mount in terms of team functioning. These multidimensional challenges underscore the importance of effective and healthy team functioning and enable professionals to work efficiently and compassionately. These challenges also illustrate the constant pressures on the team as they do their work together. Taking the time to establish a foundational understanding of team resources, generating options for managing the workload together in times of increased pressure, and trust that colleagues share goals and a vision for how patient care can be delivered will go a long way in supporting the efficacy of the service over time.

PPC TEAMS: EXAMPLES FROM THE PRACTICE WORLD

In PPC, there are both tasks and interpersonal and intrapersonal dynamics that play an important role in how patient care is delivered. However, group process is rarely thought of in terms of team function and patient care. Systems theory and group dynamics theory offer perspectives on creative approaches to teams. If we see the team as a group or system that functions dynamically in order to accomplish certain tasks, we can begin to conceptualize the process of evolution of the team. Events like episodes of conflict, growth, and relationship-building can be seen as predictable processes to be managed, rather than a crisis.

Case Example: Communication

Dusty is an 1-year-old boy with static encephalopathy and severe cerebral palsy, the result of an intracranial bleed when he was born prematurely. Dusty functions at the level of a 6-month old, able to respond to voices and touch with smiles and turning toward the stimuli. It is not clear if he is able to see. He has been hospitalized for the fourth time in 7 weeks with symptoms of gastrointestinal distress after G-tube feedings, including facial grimacing and writhing in bed. He lives in voluntary foster care as his mother, a single parent, has schizophrenia and has been unable to care for him since he was 2 months old. His mother has a history of exacerbation of her mental illness, including increased symptoms of depression when Dusty becomes ill. He has lived in the same foster home all this time, and his foster mother and biological mother have a mutually supportive and respectful relationship. His biological mother retains parental rights and decision-making authority, yet has only a basic understanding of Dusty's medical issues. His foster mother is very involved with his medical providers and coordinates his complex care. Dusty and his foster family live in a small town in a rural area 2 hours away from the medical center. There is mounting concern that Dusty is showing signs and symptoms of feeding intolerance secondary to deterioration in his overall condition. Acute illness and physical impairments have been ruled out. Dusty is slated for more tests. He is followed by the Neurology service, the GI service, and his pediatrician. The neurologist, his nurse, and the pediatrician have followed Dusty medically for his whole life. They are actively looking into additional therapies that may improve his condition and functioning in the hope that they can offer more to the families. The neurologist is very distressed about this sad turn of events, and is anxious to find a solution. The Pediatric Palliative Care Team (PPCT) has been asked by Dusty's pediatrician to see him, to make recommendations for interventions to promote his comfort, and to help identify goals for care should his condition in fact be deteriorating.

As this case description illustrates, in PPC, there are many important issues to address simultaneously. Family stability and family system integrity may be challenged by a new diagnosis, significant changes in the child's condition, or impending death. Adaptation to the complex world of specialty pediatric health care is a complex task in and of itself. There is great pressure to assimilate complex information in emotionally trying circumstances. Resources that enable the family to make choices about care for the child who is ill, other family caregiving roles, and workplace demands may be jeopardized by competing pressures at times. The perceived suffering of a child is a very compelling situation for the family and for the team. It makes sense that a team approach to care, in which individuals with diverse yet overlapping expertise, can provide the family with greater assistance than a single professional striving to help the family manage.

Like families, teams experience competing pressures from many directions. Efforts are directed at meeting family goals, undertaking complex and creative problem solving, managing multiple cases at a time, coping with a high degree of uncertainty with regard to disease trajectories and outcomes, and meeting organizational imperatives. In addition, professionals are likely to have personal commitment to their work, discipline specific priorities, deep connections with patients and families, and a desire to be professionally well-regarded by colleagues. As Dusty's case illustrated, well-intentioned individuals may struggle with what is best to do, how to support families, and how to help families understand an uncertain, changing situation. Concerns about appropriate boundaries, managing relationships so that perceived "overly involved" practitioners do not inadvertently influence decisions or care options out of misplaced concern, and efforts to avoid difficult emotions are common dynamics in pediatric palliative care situations. Social workers are uniquely trained to notice these dynamics and to advocate for the child and family needs (Jones, 2005). Collaboration with palliative care colleagues is a good way to bring out these complex issues and plan for containment of the process, heighten awareness of potential negative effects for the family and the staff, and intervene to minimize the impact of these dilemmas.

If we look at the provision of PPC as a dynamic, highly complex system or group process, then it is important to note the role of facilitation and maintaining the "meta-view," or the perspective on what is happening in the big picture in that group process. In our experience, it is uncommon for anyone to actually take on the role of evaluating group process of the team in a deliberate way. There may be no one in the role, or the team may not have identified that the role is even necessary. This can be a role that is shared among formal and informal team leaders, or handed off on a rotating basis. Social workers get "drafted" into these roles by virtue of their expertise in systems awareness and interpersonal dynamics (Jones, 2005). Social workers may find they notice unmet needs, communication gaps, interactional tensions, conflict situations, and signs of stress within a case situation, or among members of the team. It can be a source of validation to the whole team to name and define this role of tracking the group process, looking for barriers, conflicts, impediments, and a need for processing what is going on. Sometimes taking the time to clarify what is happening on a more complex level actually allows the team to move forward more constructively. There are internal or perhaps unconscious influences at work and sometimes a buildup of emotions and reactions that can affect the work of the team. These need to be named and time set aside for personal or team resolution to enable a return to productivity. Teams are routinely asked to perform with a high degree of professionalism in challenging circumstances. This may involve dealing with unresolved conflicts or underlying tensions among team members. In our experience, awareness that the entire team shares a primary commitment to the best interests of the child and family allows us to work together to address immediate needs and set our conflicts aside in order to address the immediate situation. Patterns of conflict avoidance or anxiety about addressing conflicts can also make it difficult to go back and address these concerns. Developing a team culture where mutual expectations are specified can help. One team, for example, has developed a "Team Covenant" which all staff sign on to when they join the team, agreeing to address conflict directly and seek help as needed (Haslinger Palliative Care Center, Akron Children's Hospital, as presented at CAPC National Conference, 2010; M. Farrar-Laco, personal communication, November 1, 2012). This consensus agreement is reviewed at orientation for new staff, and as a periodic reminder, that all staff members are expected to address conflicts directly, in a timely manner, and ask for assistance or mediation as needed.

Collaborative communication has been described as a helpful foundation for PPC. According to Feudtner (2007), this mode of communication can be understood in terms of participants' desires to accomplish at least five important tasks:

1. establish a common goal or set of goals;
2. exhibit mutual respect and compassion for each other;
3. develop a sufficiently complete understanding of differing perspectives;
4. assure maximum clarity and correctness of what we communicate with each other;
5. manage intrapersonal and interpersonal processes that affect how we send, receive, and process information.

Such a model can create a structure that helps clinicians discuss complex matters across different perspectives. This process of careful communication takes time and planning to accomplish. It is relies upon each team member's willingness to develop awareness of personal habits of thought, styles of processing of emotions, and managing interpersonal conflict (Feudtner, 2007). Social workers have training in these dimensions of interaction and can offer expertise to the team to advance a culture of open and collaborative communication in a context of high pressure and complex needs.

In practice, the evolution of an interprofessional team takes time and attention. As professionals from diverse disciplines grow into their roles, patterns get established as to how participants work together. This process can be conscious and planned or unconscious and accidental. It is important to be clear about what expectations team members have of each other so that patient and family care can flow efficiently and effectively. A kind of "short-hand" that can evolve among teams that enable members to understand and predict their behaviors, assessments, and opportunities for intervention, but that can only happen when the team has a chance to work together over time and with predictability.

Case Example: Collaboration

The PPCT physician and social worker were consulting on their plan for managing an end-of-life situation for a child they had been helping to care for over the last several weeks. As they discussed the situation, it became clear that they had differing expectations about how each other "should" play a role in the unfolding situation. The social worker felt the family was managing "OK" and did not need the team at the bedside. The physician felt it important to be present through the acute dying phase. As they shared their perspectives, it became clear the physician was con-cerned about potential moment to moment pain and symptom manage-ment needs that could occur as the child dies. The social worker assessed that the family was well-prepared for coping with this situation, based upon many hours of family counseling she had with them in recent weeks and knew that they had asked family to gather around for his last days. She felt the needs at this time were for the family to be together with their child with as few distractions as possible. She was interested in empower-ing the family to determine how they wanted these last precious days to go. As they learned more about each other's concerns, the social worker and physician noted they were attending to different yet critically important aspects of care for this child and family. These realizations helped diffuse tensions that had been developing, and also served to help them under-stand each other's focus and skill sets more fully.

Blacker and Deveau (2010) identify seven recommendations for effec-tive interprofessional team collaboration:

- organizational and leadership commitment to team structuring and role socialization;
- inclusion of patient and family as a part of the team (in pediatrics, this is reflected in the philosophy of "family-centered care");
- formation of interprofessional care plans that require some basic structure and agreed upon processes;
- clear articulation of each team member's role, professional competencies, and scope of practice;
- expect normal team struggles;
- ensure that opportunities exist for individual professional development;
- develop protocols and processes for information sharing, and care hand-offs with internal and external care providers.

In addition, trust in each other's roles and skills, and the knowledge that the rest of the team will provide back up and support when things get busy or difficult are important attributes. Trust evolves as team members work together, and learn each other's skills and strengths. The team will coalesce as successes and conflicts are managed in the course of work.

The size of the team may contribute to these dynamics in important ways. A small team of 2 or 3 individuals working together daily has more opportunity to develop a "group think," mutual understanding, and trust than a larger group of 12 or 20 rotating individuals, for example. The group dynamics in a smaller team are not as complex. When there is a shared vision of what the team is trying to accomplish, and how they will do that, then it becomes more likely for efficiencies to evolve, for trust to develop, and for team members to feel more satisfaction in their ability to contribute their expertise to the team's work. These general principles underscore the importance that the PPC team is created to have the structure, room for process, and support necessary to develop a different way of operating within the health care system to deliver specialty-level palliative care (Blacker & Deveau, 2010; Meier & Beresford, 2008). The needs that families describe for continuity, compassionate care, knowledgeable caregivers who understand their child's disease and their family challenges, and good communication are best addressed by a skilled and effective team that is uniquely situated within the health care system to respond to challenges. Advanced care planning is a particularly important area in which good team dynamics can make a difference. Communication about this often occurs over time and includes both complex medical information and psychological processing. Effective collaboration among the team members and with the family can result in a good decision-making process, good communication of the plan, and also serve to reassure the family that a good process was followed.

Communication becomes a vital task and strategy for fostering positive team collaboration. The quality of communication necessary to facilitate creative problem solving at a high level under rapidly changing circumstances and great emotional pressures is key to effective planning and safe patient care delivery. Frequent communication of facts, assessments, ideas, preferences, and feedback is essential. The frequency, depth, range, and quality of communication can make a critical difference in how care is delivered, and so has a significant effect on patient and family safety, quality of life, and satisfaction.

Case Example: Team Member Relationships

A social worker who had worked on the PPC team for many years and so was very seasoned in both the specialty practice, the organization, and the team's dynamics was speaking to a physician who was new to the team, and had moved from another state and so was also new to the organization. As they discussed how they might approach a case situation, the doctor expressed that she was not aware that social workers' training included reflection upon the use of self in interactions with clients. This led to an interesting discussion of their diverse training experiences, and how they had received very different messages in their training about what to do with personal reactions to client or patient situations. Both came away from this spontaneous sharing with a newly expanded idea of how the other came to their particular perspective on their individual role in patient care and expectations for themselves.

As our (the authors) large team has evolved over a period of years, we have observed specific tension points that occur with predictability. When our patient care load grew, had staffing shortages, and lost and added team members, we have struggled. The pressures to manage high patient care demands can be at odds with the care and attention needed to adequately mentor new staff into their role on the team. Institutional changes can also challenge resources and expectations for the team. In our experience, the evolution of our team has not been a straight line from innocence to wisdom. It is probably more realistic to view team dynamics as constantly changing and unfolding. As we have addressed ongoing and emerging issues, at times, it has felt like taking "two steps forward, one step back." Confounding factors like compassion fatigue and burnout among team members can also complicate the picture. We may overestimate the frequency of difficult situations, for example, or fall into patterns of attributing "never" and "always" to concerns. In traditional group process models, we learned to expect "forming, storming norming, and performing" as stages of development in progress. (Tuckman, 1965/2001) For teams, we may need to consider something more like: forming, storming, norming, performing, reforming and storming again, then norming and performing, until the next time we are forming again.

As colleagues were added to the team, the assumptions about how we would work together were never discussed or affirmed with one another. As a result, conflicts escalated and the team needed to "step back" and address those and clarify expectations going forward. It was hard for the team to make time for these complicated discussions (Stone, Patton, & Heen, 1999). The busy pace of work and also a natural desire to avoid conflict proved to be barriers. The processing of team dynamics needed attention in order for us to be able to work together as effectively as we could. Again, this is typically a process that is not often actively facilitated and so it is easy for these discussions to not occur and for conflicts to be "swept under the rug." It is important to have a structure for checking in on the team's health and functioning in these important areas, including accountability for the process.

CONCLUSION

It is easy to forget that health care providers (and family members), have little control over an individual child's illness course. We "hope for the best and prepare for the rest." Flexibility, creativity, and a healthy respect for what we cannot control are qualities that contribute to sustainability for individual clinicians, and for the team as a whole. Social work values and skills that include insight into systems, and facilitation of group dynamics and process, communication skills like clarification and reframing, conflict resolution and mediation, respect for the value of diversity, and the interaction of parts for the good of the whole can make important contributions to effective pediatric palliative care team dynamics. By fostering effective collaboration, advocating for team resources, explicating the dynamics in play, and modeling brave and principled approaches to conflict and problem solving, social workers are in a position to provide important leadership in this challenging and exciting new field of palliative care.

RESOURCES

- Center to Advance Palliative Care (CAPC): Palliative Care Program Development Training, Resources, and Tools: http://www.capc.org
- National Hospice and Palliative Care Organization: Online Curriculum for Pediatric Palliative Care, Pediatric Palliative Care Standards: http://www.NHPCO.Org/Pediatrics
- ELNEC-Pediatrics—Training for Nurses in Pediatric Palliative Care: http://www.ucdmc.ucdavis.edu/cne/classes/pediatric_elnec.html
- EPEC-Pediatrics—End of Life and Palliative Care Training: http://www.epec.net
- Strategies for Managing Change: http://www.strategies-for-managing-change.com/
- Team Stepps Training: http://teamstepps.ahrq.gov

REFERENCES

Abramson, J. S., & Mizrahi, T. (2003). Understanding collaboration between social workers and physicians: Application of a typology. *Social Work in Health Care, 37*(2), 71–100.

Blacker, S., & Deveau, C. (2010). Social work and interprofessional collaboration in palliative care. *Progress in Palliative Care, 18*(4), 237–243.

Feudtner, C. (2007). Collaborative communication in pediatric palliative care: A foundation of problem-solving and decision-making. *Pediatric Clinics of North America, 54*, 583–607.

Jones, B. (2005.) Pediatric palliative and end-of-life care: The role of social work in pediatric oncology. *Journal of Social Work in End-of-Life & Palliative Care, 1*(4), 35–62.

Meier, D., & Beresford, L. (2008). The palliative care team. *Journal of Palliative Medicine, 11*(5), 677–681.

O'Connor, M., & Fisher, C. (2011). Exploring the dynamics of interdisciplinary palliative care teams in providing psychosocial care: "Everybody thinks that everybody can do it and they can't." *Journal of Palliative Medicine, 4*(2), 191–196.

Stone, D., Patton, B. M., & Heen, S. (1999). *Difficult conversations: How to discuss what matters most.* New York, NY: Penguin Books.

Tuckman, B. (2001). Developmental sequence in small groups. *Group Facilitation: A Research and Applications Journal, 3*, 66–81. (Reprinted from *Psychological Bulletin, 63*, 384–399, by the American Psychological Association, 1965)

Youngwerth, J., & Twaddle, M. (2011). Cultures of interdisciplinary teams: How to foster good dynamics. *Journal of Palliative Medicine, 14*(5), 650–654. doi:10.1089/jpm.2010.0395

Zimmerman, J., & Dabelko, H. I. (2007). Collaborative models of patient care. *Social Work in Health Care, 44*(4), 33–47.

Palliative Care in the Pediatric ICU: Challenges and Opportunities for Family-Centered Practice

ARDITH DOORENBOS

Department of Biobehavioral Nursing & Health Systems, School of Nursing, University of Washington, Seattle, Washington, USA

TARYN LINDHORST

School of Social Work, University of Washington, Seattle, Washington, USA

HELENE STARKS

Department of Bioethics and Humanities, School of Medicine, University of Washington, Seattle, Washington, USA

EUGENE AISENBERG

School of Social Work, University of Washington, Seattle, Washington, USA

J. RANDALL CURTIS

Department of Medicine, Division of Pulmonary and Critical Care Medicine, School of Medicine, University of Washington, Seattle, Washington, USA

ROSS HAYS

Center for Child Health, Behavior and Development, Seattle Children's Research Institute, and Department of Rehabilitative Medicine, School of Medicine, University of Washington, Seattle, Washington, USA

The culture of pediatric intensive care units (PICUs) is focused on curative or life-prolonging treatments for seriously ill children. We present empirically-based approaches to family-centered palliative care that can be applied in PICUs. Palliative care in these settings is framed by larger issues related to the context of care in PICUs, the stressors experienced by families, and challenges to palliative care philosophy within this environment. Innovations from research on family-centered communication practices in adult ICU settings provide a framework for development of palliative care in PICUs and suggest avenues for social work support of critically ill children and their families.

Historically, the goal of patient care in pediatric intensive care units (PICU)[1] has been to do everything medically possible to cure a child's illness or prolong life. Childhood deaths are decreasing in the United States, with 53,552 deaths or 2.2% among children aged 0–19 years in 2005, which is significantly less than in 2000 (Martin et al., 2008). Yet, for some seriously or terminally ill children, the curative focus of the PICU will not prevent death. Pediatric deaths most typically are a result of congenital birth defects, cancers, traumatic injuries, and genetic or neurological disorders (Sands, Manning, Vyas, & Rashid, 2009). When curative therapies are no longer appropriate, or in cases where the outcome for seriously ill children is highly uncertain but could realistically end in death, PICU staff members face a transition in care to one that addresses the end-of-life issues. They must prioritize the physical and emotional comfort of the child and family while balancing continued treatment intended to prolong life (Friebert, 2009). In many cases, this transition, if it happens at all, comes very late in the trajectory of a child's serious illness and often only after every possible medical intervention has been pursued at length (Carter, Hubble, & Weise, 2006). The desire to continue aggressive care is supported by clinicians and families alike, especially when intensive interventions sometimes do succeed and offer a reason to invest in the hope and possibility of continued therapy (Byrne et al., 2011).

In the fast-paced, aggressive, care-focused environment of the PICU, the initiation and delivery of palliative care has unique challenges that require effective communication between the family and the health care team about their collective understanding of the possibilities for intervention, the likely and desired outcomes given the child's illness and capacities, and the goals of care for the child and family (Hays et al., 2006). Because of competing demands that keep the focus of care on the diagnosis and treatment of the child's illness, the in-depth assessment of the child and family's beliefs, values, and understanding of the medical implications of the illness or condition is often not the main concern within the context of the highly technological and procedure-focused environment of the PICU. Social workers can be key players in facilitating communication because of their training in culturally sensitive assessment, expertise in interaction and group process, life course development, family systems and dynamics theories, and their role as liaisons between clinicians and families (Fineberg, 2010). The purpose of this article is to provide information on empirically based approaches to family-centered palliative care which can be applied in a PICU setting. Any effort to introduce palliative care into PICUs is framed by larger issues related to the context of care in these units, the stresses experienced by families with a critically ill child, and the challenges to palliative care within this environment. Recent innovations from research on family-centered communication practices in adult ICU settings provide a framework for further development of palliative care in pediatric intensive care, and suggest avenues for social work support of critically ill children and their families.

THE CONTEXT OF CARE IN PEDIATRIC INTENSIVE CARE UNITS

Every year at least 200 children per 100,000 require hospitalization in PICUs because of serious illness (Shudy et al., 2006). Approximately 90% of pediatric deaths in the hospital occur in neonatal and pediatric intensive care units (Carter et al., 2004; Field & Behrman, 2003). These settings are characterized by their intensive technological focus on life-saving procedures such as the use of mechanical breathing assistance (ventilation), intensive intravenous (IV) administration of medications, and artificial hydration and nutrition supplementation. Most deaths in the PICU are preceded by withdrawal of life-prolonging medical therapy, most typically mechanical ventilation (Sands et al., 2009; Shudy et al. 2006), the removal of these can result in death from respiratory arrest within moments to hours.

In addition to the medical acuity of the children seen in PICU settings, the organization of care in these units is also complex, especially from a family's perspective. Families and patients in these settings interact with multiple professional caregivers including physicians, nurses, pharmacists, nutritionists, child life specialists, respiratory therapists, social workers and depending on the child's condition, specialists from medical disciplines such as nephrology, cardiology, pulmonology, and oncology. Many PICUs are located in teaching hospitals where in addition to attending physicians, families may also encounter residents and fellows who rotate through the unit on a weekly or monthly basis. In the course of a 24-hour period, families may interact with dozens of medical professionals each of whom has some responsibility for the care of their child. They then may encounter a substantially new set of caregivers the next day. Care may not be well coordinated among these multiple services and disciplines and communication may be fragmented, thus affecting the family's ability to access appropriate information and to make informed decisions regarding the care of their child.

While daily rounds in which the interdisciplinary professional team discusses the medical indications for treatment of the child are routine in PICUs, these conversations may or may not include family members. Even when family members are physically present, the usual purpose of the rounds is to review highly technical medical findings that are typically outside of most family members' understanding. Rarely are families invited into the conversation or given explanations about what each lab value, medication, or machine setting indicates. As a result, families often face challenges in obtaining information about their child's condition and care needs that is understandable to them. This difficulty becomes even more pronounced when medical teams are caring for children and families with limited English language skills. When interpreters are available, they usually have to be requested in advance, so emergent changes in a child's condition may not be communicated to family members.

In response to efforts to improve care in PICUs, several changes have been recommended to include families more directly in the care of their children, drawing on practice principles derived from models of "family-centered care," which is broadly focused on building partnerships between families and health care providers when caring for critically ill patients (Cooley, 2001; Frazier, Frazier, & Warren, 2009; Johnson, 2000; Johnson & Eichner, 2003; National Association of Children's Hospitals and Related Institutions [NACHRI], 2009). Truog, Meyer, and Burns (2006) have identified six domains that are central to family-centered care: (a) support of the family unit; (b) communication with the child and family about treatment goals and plans; (c) ethics and shared decision making; (d) relief of pain and other symptoms; (e) continuity of care; and (f) grief and bereavement support. A family-centered approach requires a core commitment to including patients and families as respected members of the health care team, and communicating with them in ways which elicit patient and family values, needs, and preferences (Frazier et al., 2009). For example, in response to parental concerns to have ongoing access to their child, many units have made provisions for parents to "room in" with their children in a more aesthetically appealing environment, rather than allowing only brief visitations each hour. These rooming-in arrangements support positive attachment and provide emotional security for the child. Rooming in can reduce the stress of travel for the parent and the stress of the hospital stay for the child and parent. Also, research suggests that such arrangements in pediatric care units can reduce parental stress caused by changes in the parental role that can occur during pediatric hospitalizations (Smith, Hefley, & Anand, 2007).

The Society of Critical Care Medicine (SCCM) has developed clinical practice guidelines for the support of the patients and families in adult, pediatric, and neonatal ICUs (Davidson et al., 2007). These evidence-based guidelines address family psychosocial needs by recommending shared decision making; routine care conferences with families to explain the patient's medical condition and determine mutually agreed upon goals of care; cultural and spiritual support for patient and family; and family support before, during, and after a death. These guidelines recognize the need for interprofessional practice, and highlight the role that social workers can play in each of these areas. Yet, as discussed below, changing ICU practice remains an ongoing challenge despite advances in the recognition of the importance of family-centered care (Balluffi et al., 2004; Contro, Larson, Scofield, Sourkes, & Cohen, 2002; Carlet et al., 2004).

STRESSORS FOR FAMILIES WITH A CRITICALLY ILL CHILD

The serious illness and death of a child is one of the most disruptive events in a family's life experience, especially when the family is raising young children (Hooyman & Kramer, 2006). Research has documented that parents often have intense grief after the death of a child. Death in the PICU is often unexpected by parents who are hoping for recovery with use of aggressive therapies (Meert, Thurston, & Thomas, 2001). Complicated grief was found in 59% of parents whose child had died in the PICU, 6 months after the death (Meert et al., 2010). The majority of parents (74%) report having experienced some resolution of their grief after the death of a child (Kreicbergs et al., 2007); however, parents with unresolved grief reported significantly worsening psychological health and physical health compared with those who have experienced some resolution of their grief (Lannen, Wolfe, Prigerson, Onelov, & Kreicbergs, 2008). Parental stress may also limit the emotional and physical availability of parents for other children in the home, particularly in response to sibling fears, concerns, and anxieties. For example, the more depressed or distressed the parent in dealing with the serious illness of a child, the less able the parent will be to act as a buffer for siblings; in such circumstances, the sibling may refrain from disclosing to parents or revealing emotions out of a strong desire not to burden other family members or add to others' distress (Aisenberg, 2006).

Parents not only are caregivers for their children, but also are "second-order patients" themselves who require attention from PICU staff (Rait & Lederberg, 1989). The PICU is an emotionally charged environment that places major demands on patients and family caregivers and can have negative effects on their short- and long-term psychosocial outcomes (Azoulay et al., 2001; Board & Ryan-Wenger, 2002; Contro et al., 2002; Meert et al., 2001; Studdert et al., 2003). For example, Balluffi and colleagues (2004) assessed the prevalence of two anxiety disorders among parents caring for a child in a PICU. During the initial period of the PICU admission, about one third of the parents met symptom criteria for Acute Stress Disorder (ASD).

Four months after the PICU discharge, 21% of parents met symptom criteria for Post-Traumatic Stress Disorder (PTSD). Nearly all parents experienced one or more of four types of symptoms associated with PTSD—including feelings of dissociation, re-experiencing the stressful event, avoidance of the stressful event, or hyper-arousal. ASD rates were higher among parents who worried their child might die and for whom the admission was unexpected (Balluffi et al., 2004), both of which are characteristic of children who may benefit from palliative care consultation.

Adding another layer of stress for parents are the conflicts that can arise regarding care decisions in the PICU. These decisions are typically made by parents because their children are cognitively and/or legally not able to make autonomous choices about the kind of care they receive. This structural difference between adult and pediatric care requires that communication in a pediatric environment be focused on family system functioning, not just the desires and goals of the patient. Perception of support is a key determinant in psychosocial outcomes for parents—including support given by clinicians (Melnyk, Feinstein, & Fairbanks, 2006; Truog et al., 2006), PICU and other hospital staff, and family or friends (Briller, Meert, Schim, Thurston, & Kabel, 2009; Meert, Briller, Thurston, & Schim, 2008). However, in the only study specifically focused on the PICU setting, Studdert and colleagues (2003) found serious disagreements in over one-half of the cases where children spent more than eight days in intensive care. Conflicts between the medical team and family were the most common (60%) and were associated with poor communication (48%); unavailability of a parent/guardian (39%); disagreements over the child's care plan (39%); coping problems (21%); dysfunctional families (12%); conflicts about decision making (9%); and young parents (6%). Intrateam conflicts were also present in over one third of cases, but intrafamily conflict was rare, occurring in only 2% of families, and most often associated with a disagreement over the care plan. Where there is conflict between staff and families, ethics consultations have been shown to be beneficial in adult environments (Schneiderman et al., 2003).

The needs of families may not be recognized by the physicians charged with the care of seriously ill children because of different perspectives regarding which processes and outcomes are most important in PICU care. For example, one study found that families valued clear communication and compassionate support at the end of life more than pain management or length of stay; however, physicians prioritized technical aspects of pain management and length of stay as the most important factors (Mack et al., 2005). Meyer, Burns, Griffith, and Truog (2002) reported that over half of families in the PICU considered the possibility of withdrawing life-prolonging interventions before any such discussions were initiated by the medical team, and up to 25% of parents reported that, in retrospect, they would have made decisions differently than those that were recommended by staff concerning their child's care. Unfortunately, because of the power differentials and structures of the PICU settings, families remain at a disadvantage in negotiating care in the PICU. The PICU is still a very technologically focused environment and has yet to become a family-friendly place despite a decade of study and dissemination of the concept of family-centered care in pediatrics. In this context, social workers can exercise crucial leadership to facilitate and enhance communication between parents and members of the medical team. Trained in addressing crisis and loss, social workers can also facilitate communication across the multiple services and members of the interdisciplinary palliative care team that are engaged in the care of the hospitalized child.

PALLIATIVE CARE AT END OF LIFE IN THE PICU

The goal of palliative care is to improve quality of life by relieving pain and other distressing symptoms for patients and families facing life-threatening illness (World Health Organization, 2010) and to assist patients and families in decision making about end-of-life care. Palliative care is family-centered support that includes physical, emotional, and spiritual comfort which is best provided by a multidisciplinary team that includes social workers, physicians, nurses, chaplains, and other health care professionals (Friedman, Hilden & Powaski, 2005; Teno et al., 2004). Patients are typically eligible for palliative care services from the time of diagnosis through death and into bereavement (Field & Behrman, 2003; Friedman et al., 2005); thus the mission of and services offered by palliative care can extend far beyond the typical 6-month prognosis used to determine eligibility for hospice by Medicare and most other private insurances in the United States. In addition, it is important to conceptualize palliative care as broader than end-of-life care. Although palliative care should be a component of end-of-life care, palliative care also includes care earlier in the disease trajectory focused on identifying the goals of care—including patient and family support for physical, emotional and spiritual issues that arise in the context of a potentially life-limiting illness (Curtis & Rubenfeld, 2005). Hospital-based palliative care teams often function in a more consultative role, especially for the critically ill, rather than directly providing ongoing nursing or other direct patient care services. However, some palliative care programs are integrated with hospice teams and more direct patient care is provided. During the past decade, pediatric palliative care teams have grown in number. Hospital-based pediatric palliative care teams deal with a greater diversity of medical conditions and duration of survival than palliative care teams caring for adult patients (Feudtner et al., 2011).

Both families and clinicians share the hope and expectation that ill or injured children will improve with aggressive care, so it is common that the unquestioned goal of care is to pursue every available option in the PICU. The desire to preserve and prolong life in the PICU has a heightened poignancy due the youth of the patients and the feeling that they have not yet had their lives to live. In this respect, the PICU may have a greater focus on cure in contrast to the more varied strategies and goals that might be considered for older adults in ICUs. As a result, palliative care in pediatric intensive care settings has been slower to develop than in adult ICUs where the patient mix often includes a substantial number of elderly adults who may be facing the end of life as a normal and expected part of the human life course. Barriers to good palliative care from family perspectives include a primary focus on curative treatments (Carter et al., 2006), dealing with a complex team of clinicians who are often not communicating consistent information, and the perception that decisions must be made quickly without enough time to absorb and act on changing situations (Briller et al., 2009).

Integrating palliative care into the PICU setting can be challenging for both logistical and provider-oriented reasons. Studies of death in PICUs suggest that even though some children are in the PICU for months, the median length of stay is around one week (Carter et al., 2004). Although one week is too short for optimal delivery of palliative care, even this short time can be used to incorporate palliative care consultation, particularly about goals of care and end-of-life decision making. However, children with serious chronic conditions may have multiple admissions to PICUs over the course of their illness. In these circumstances, families may benefit from palliative care that is offered in a more episodic fashion.

Communicating the prognosis of seriously or terminally ill children is a delicate process that can be more difficult in the milieu of the PICU. The uncertainty surrounding prognosis for many pediatric conditions poses another logistical issue in recognizing that end-of-life concerns should be addressed. For example, organ transplantation, an increasingly common category of ICU care, represents the entire spectrum of outcomes from full recovery to death. An infant in need of a heart transplant may die before the transplant can be obtained, or if a donor heart is found and transplanted successfully, the child may have a normal life expectancy. Many pediatric conditions have unclear trajectories, and given the focus on curative treatment, it can be difficult to raise the possibility of death when continued life and improved health are the hoped for outcomes (Byrne et al., 2011).

Health care professionals trained in critical or intensive care often feel personal discomfort when discussing quality-of-life or end-of-life issues and may therefore avoid or delay important conversations (Contro, Larson, Scofield, Sourkes, & Cohen, 2004; Hinds, Schum, Baker, & Wolfe, 2005). However, delaying such difficult conversations can result in missed opportunities for identification and resolution of emotional issues and for healing within the family (Hutton, 2002). The prevailing style of clinician communication to family members is typically a physiologic systems approach, focusing on ventilator settings, incremental changes in laboratory values, and other highly technical data. This approach usually does not directly address the child's chances for survival or future level of functioning. For example, 70% of families in one study felt they had been well-informed about their child's chances for survival (Meyer et al., 2002), yet only 14% of parents felt they had been adequately informed about their child's deteriorating physical condition as death approached (Davies & Connaughty, 2002). Frequently, PICU clinicians engage in frank discussions about prognosis only after they judge the future quality of life as unacceptable, at which point they use this information to suggest discontinuation of life-prolonging interventions (Meyer, Ritholz, Burns, & Truog, 2006).

Several studies have examined the health care providers' comfort and confidence levels in providing pediatric palliative care in the PICU. In general, the staff of PICUs felt less comfortable providing psychosocial care compared to other aspects of care (Jones et al., 2007). Additionally, confidence in providing palliative care was significantly higher among physicians and nurses who had eight years or more of experience in the PICU (Jones et al., 2007). These findings suggest that palliative care conversations are difficult for the clinicians directly engaged in the care of critically ill children in pediatric intensive care settings. Social workers who have training in discussing uncomfortable issues can help initiate these conversations when they are aware that there is uncertainty about the child's potential for recovery.

INTEGRATING FAMILY-CENTERED COMMUNICATION INTO PICU SETTINGS

Excellent communication skills are essential in the PICU setting because of the high-stakes decisions; critical informational needs of families; and the numerous potential differences in cultural beliefs, understanding, values, and preferences between clinicians and families (Azoulay et al., 2001; Contro et al., 2002; Hinds et al., 2005; Meyer et al., 2006). Family-centered practice recommends that the appropriate role for family members for decision making about goals of care and discussion of end-of-life issues is generally that of shared decision making in concert with the clinicians (Carlet et al., 2004). However, it is important to realize that there is a spectrum of preferred decision-making roles for family members that can extend from decisions being made exclusively by family members on one end of the spectrum to families who would prefer to delegate decisions to clinicians on the other end (Heyland et al., 2003). Furthermore, research suggests that family members' risk for psychological symptoms after a death in the ICU is higher if their preferred decision-making role does not match their actual decision-making role (Gries et al., 2010). Clinicians should develop skills to match the clinicians' and families' role with families' needs and preferred role (Curtis & White, 2008; White, Malvar, Karr, Lo, & Curtis, 2010).

Parents have reported that they prefer for detailed medical information to be integrated into a larger context so that they can understand individual treatments, changes in status, and decision options within a "big picture" perspective of their child's overall care (Meyer et al., 2006). While clinical data are important, many families prioritize quality of life in their decision making. Unfortunately, quality of life issues are rarely addressed by providers until the child is in an acute crisis. A "take it as it comes" approach to discussing trajectories of illness may be the desired approach of some families, and may be necessary when the potential effects of treatment are difficult to predict (Byrne et al., 2011). In the absence of anticipatory guidance, families live without a full understanding of the possible choices they may have in response to acute episodes of chronic conditions. For example, with guidance, the family of a child with relapsed cancer, may be able to anticipate when hospitalizations are likely to occur and then plan family activities to maximize the child's experiences when she or he is home. Children and families might prioritize their quality of life at home over time in the hospital if they understood the prognosis and treatment options. However, in the absence of conversations about possible trajectories of the condition, planning is more difficult and decision making may happen in the context of a crisis, precisely when families would prefer it not to occur.

Studies from adult ICUs provide some insight into specific tools that may help clinicians improve communication with family members. One is the use of family care conferences to share information and determine the goals of care for the patient (Fineberg, Kawashima, & Asch, 2011). Care conferences can be formal meetings with agendas, or happen informally at the bedside of the patient. Typically, they cover content that is described in Table 1 and are usually led by a designated member, often the palliative care team member and/or the patient's primary physician. The format of these meetings usually includes preconference planning for the optimal use of the conference time; opening, information sharing, and moderation of discussion at the care conference; closing summary of important goals and decisions; and follow-up post-care conference to answer any emerging questions (Ambuel, 2000). Family care conferences offer the opportunity to "unpack" unfamiliar medical terms and diagnoses; for example, using the term "allow natural death" rather than "do not resuscitate" when suggesting not using extraordinary lifesaving measures (Jones et al., 2008). A skilled facilitator of these meetings will ensure not just that this information is provided by the medical team, but that the family can state their understanding in their own terms. The planning, facilitation, and follow-up to family care conferences enhance clinician-patient-family relationships, communication, and care coordination—which builds trust, the sense of being heard, and access to information and support (Meyer et al., 2006). When a standardized family conference was coupled with the use of the "VALUE" mnemonic for improving communication (see Figure 1), a randomized trial found that family

TABLE 1 Typical Information Shared in a Family Care Conference

Introductions, reasons and goals for the conference	• Goals should be ascertained from both patient/family members and professional care providers
Medical condition	• Brief history • Current treatments • Current symptoms • Recent changes
Prognostic information	• Anticipated prognosis with and without disease-directed treatments • Likely level of functioning under each scenario
Patient/Family psychosocial information	• How patient and family define quality of life • Family communication dynamics • Current stressors • Developmental issues of patient and/or family
Decision making	• Obtain consensus on decisions to be made • Obtain consensus on treatment decisions • Anticipate future decisions that may need to be made

Note. Adapted from Weissman, Quill, and Arnold (2010a, 2010b).

members reported reduced symptoms of anxiety, depression, and PTSD (Lautrette et al., 2007).

Other studies have identified specific components of clinician communication that were related to enhanced family functioning—including having a private place for family communication, consistent communication by all

---

VALUE: 5 -step Approach to Improving

Communication in ICU with Families

• V… Value family statements

• A… Acknowledge family emotions

• L… Listen to the family

• U… Understand the patient as a person

• E… Elicit family questions

FIGURE 1 VALUE Mnemonic for Improving Communication with Families (Reprinted with permission from Curtis & White, 2008).

members of the team (Pochard et al., 2001), and empathic statements by clinicians (Fineberg et al., 2011; Selph, Shiang, Engelberg, Curtis, & White, 2008). Research has demonstrated that physicians often talk the longest and are more likely to determine the topics covered in patient care conferences (Fine, Reid, Shengelia, & Adelman, 2010), yet families report more satisfaction when clinicians spend more time listening and less time talking (McDonagh et al., 2004). Other features of clinician communication associated with improved family experiences include assurances the patient will not be abandoned prior to death; that every effort will be made to treat physical, emotional, and spiritual suffering of the patient; and that family decisions are explicitly supported (Stapleton, Engelberg, Wenrich, Goss, & Curtis, 2006).

Communication interventions have reduced family stress in the ICU by addressing informational needs, providing emotional support, creating a collaborative environment for clinicians and families, and reducing the potential for conflict and misunderstanding (Burns et al., 2003; Curtis et al., 2005; Tulsky, 2005). Components of successful interventions include being proactive (Hays et al., 2006); being collaborative by bringing care teams and families together in facilitated care conferences (Curtis et al., 2005); and using a structured communication process to systematically discuss and document the patient's medical condition, the patient and family's preferences, definitions of quality of life, and any contextual factors that are important to decision making (Hays et al., 2006; Jonsen, Siegler, & Winslade, 2002). When implemented proactively, communication interventions empower families and create opportunities to exchange information and understanding about the medical circumstances, acknowledge and address family emotions, explore patient and family preferences, explain the process of decision making, and affirm nonabandonment by the clinical team (Hays et al., 2006; West, Engelberg, Wenrich, & Curtis, 2005).

IMPLICATIONS FOR SOCIAL WORK PRACTICE

Social workers have a crucial responsibility to facilitate the patient and family's understanding of the medical condition and the health care team's nonjudgmental understanding of the family within the pediatric intensive care setting. Social workers provide guidance to both the multidisciplinary team and to families on psychosocial, cultural, and spiritual issues. They facilitate communication between the multidisciplinary team and family; provide support and counseling to family members; obtain concrete financial resources; coordinate care delivery; and advocate for family's needs, choices, and desires (Jones et al., 2007). Social workers may also bear witness to suffering, provide spiritual support, pain and symptom management, and bereavement follow-up; and deal with ethical issues such as truth-telling and discontinuation of treatment (Browning, 2004; Csikai & Chaitin, 2006). Social work is well situated to provide a unique and essential contribution to the multidisciplinary pediatric palliative care team with its emphasis on fostering self-determination, empowerment, and social support (Raymer & Reese, 2004).

Social work education provides an excellent foundation for addressing complex family dynamics that may emerge as a result of the medical crisis, or be continuations of family problems or coping patterns that now intersect with the critical care decisions that have to be made for a seriously ill child. Information needs to be shared with the patient and family members according to their developmental ability and in age-appropriate terms (Christ, 2000). Children who have been told about the impending death of a loved one and who are encouraged to ask questions and express feelings cope more successfully and report fewer depressive symptoms than children without this knowledge and opportunity (Sahler, 2000). Conversely, withholding information or excluding children from discussions and preparations for these important life events in the name of "protection" can lead to adverse outcomes. For example, not including siblings in conversations about the medical condition of their ill sister or brother may further isolate well children and leave them to their own imaginations in which they experience exaggerated feelings or self-blame for events that are clearly outside their control (Aisenberg, 2006).

Social work's expertise in managing communication with culturally diverse groups is also an asset to palliative care in the PICU. While talking about one's problems may be understood as therapeutic in Euro-centric cultures, not all families may be comfortable sharing personal information or information about family members. Aisenberg (2006) notes, for example, that other-centered or "allocentric oriented cultures such as Latino and Asian/Pacific Islander cultures may have more boundaries around what is private information and what is community information in effort to save face" (p. 579). Cultural differences in health beliefs in terms of causes of conditions and where power for healing lies may also affect decision making and communication in pediatric intensive care settings (MacLachlan, 2007).

Organizationally, two approaches can be taken to strengthen social work's role in the provision of family-centered palliative care in PICUs (Meier & Beresford, 2008). First, PICU social workers can receive further training on how to integrate the precepts of palliative care into their practice. While Jones and colleagues (2007) found that social workers in PICUs felt well-prepared to counsel parents, provide emotional support, and facilitate access to medical information, they were less comfortable with discussions about the transition from curative to palliative care, advocacy around symptom management and pain control, and providing education about disease progression. Specialized mentoring and training for PICU social workers in palliative care philosophies and techniques could help unit social workers to recognize when palliative care is appropriate and provide guidance in its implementation. This approach may also help with continuity of care as families work with one social worker over the course of their hospitalization. A complementary strategy is to increase the presence of specialized palliative care programs within PICU settings. Social workers frequently serve as members of the multidisciplinary palliative care team, and can contribute specific expertise in family communication within the team and the PICU setting as well as among the medical team members themselves. Often palliative care services are staffed in such a way that allows smaller caseloads and more intensive family contact than may be possible for a PICU social worker who is responsible for all social work services on the unit (Meier & Beresford, 2008). The advantage of this approach is that social workers with specialized expertise can help families anticipate, recognize, and plan for changes that are associated with the worsening of the child's condition.

As palliative care has been most strongly developed in adult settings, it will be important for palliative care clinicians to become familiar with the differences that occur in pediatric settings. Unique psychosocial concerns and needs emerge for families when serious illness occurs in a life phase that is developmentally "off time," especially where there is a need to discuss end-of-life concerns (Hooyman & Kramer, 2006). Children with potentially life-threatening conditions face highly uncertain clinical paths—sometimes their illness ends in death, but in other instances, full recovery may be possible (Byrne et al., 2011). Managing this degree of uncertainty in the context of differing developmental expectations differentiates pediatric palliative care from palliative care for elderly adults or adults with illnesses that have known trajectories. Social workers trained in empathic communication, systems theory, and family development are in a unique position to provide important leadership in promoting age-appropriate and family-centered communication and decision making.

CONCLUSIONS

Enhancement and integration of palliative care represents an important opportunity for improvement in the PICU. Integration of the principles and practice of palliative care into the pediatric ICU setting is an opportunity for incorporating family-centered care and enhancing communication between family members and the interdisciplinary clinical team. Social workers are some of the most highly trained professional in the PICU in the art and science of communication. Families value communication above all else when their child is critically ill (Meyer et al., 2002). Because of this, social workers are poised to excel as leaders in the adoption of palliative care in the PICU setting.

NOTE

1. In hospitals which have intensive care units, these can focus on the general population, which includes the adult and pediatric population (ICUs), general pediatric care (PICUs), neonatal intensive care (NICUs), or cardiac care (CICUs). In this article, we will use the term PICU to refer to all three pediatric specific sites, understanding that there are some differences between the kinds of patients and structures found in each unit.

REFERENCES

Aisenberg, E. (2006). Grief work with elementary and middle school students: Walking with hope when a child grieves. In C. Franklin, M. B. Harris, & P. Allen-Meares (Eds.), *The school services sourcebook: A guide for social workers, counselors and mental health professionals* (pp. 577–585). New York, NY: Oxford University Press.

Ambuel, B. (2000). Conducting a family conference. *Principles & Practice of Supportive Oncology, 3*, 1–12.

Azoulay, E., Pochard, F., Chevret, S., Lemaire, F., Mokhtari, M., LeGall, J. R., … French FAMIREA Group. (2001). Meeting the needs of intensive care unit patient families: A multicenter study. *American Journal of Respiratory Critical Care Medicine, 163*, 135–139.

Balluffi, A., Kassam-Adams, N., Kazak, A., Tucker, M., Dominguez, T., & Halfaer, M. (2004). Traumatic stress in parents of children admitted to the pediatric intensive care unit. *Pediatric Critical Care Medicine, 5*, 547–553.

Board, R., & Ryan-Wenger, N. (2002). Long-term effects of pediatric intensive care unit hospitalization on families with young children. *Heart and Lung, 31*, 53–66.

Briller, S. H., Meert, K. L., Schim, S. M., Thurston, C., & Kabel, A. (2009). Examining the needs of bereaved parents in the pediatric intensive care unit: A qualitative study. *Death Studies, 33*, 712–740.

Browning, D. (2004). Fragments of love: Explorations in the ethnography of suffering and professional caregiving. In J. Berzoff & P. R. Silverman (Eds.), *Living with dying: A handbook for end-of-life healthcare practitioners* (pp. 21–42). New York, NY: Columbia University Press.

Burns, J. P., Mello, M. M., Studdert, D. M., Puopolo, A. L., Truog, R. D., & Brennan, T. A. (2003). Results of a clinical trial on care improvement for the critically ill. *Critical Care Medicine, 31*, 2107–2117.

Byrne, M., Tresgallo, M., Saroyan, J., Granowetter, L., Valoy, G., & Schecter, W. (2011). Qualitative analysis of consults by a pediatric advanced care team during its first year of service. *American Journal of Hospice and Palliative Medicine, 28*, 109–117.

Carlet, J., Thijs, L. G., Antonelli, M., Cassell, J., Cox, P., Hill, N., … Thompson, B. T. (2004). Challenges in end-of-life care in the ICU: Statement of the 5th International Consensus Conference in Critical Care: Brussels, Belgium, April 2003. *Intensive Care Medicine, 30*, 770–784.

Carter, B. S., Howenstein, M., Gilmer, M. J., Throop, P., France, D., & Whitlock, J. (2004). Circumstances surrounding the deaths of hospitalized children: Opportunities for pediatric palliative care. *Pediatrics, 114*, e361– e366.

Carter, B. S., Hubble, C., & Weise, K. L. (2006). Palliative medicine in neonatal and pediatric intensive care. *Child and Adolescent Psychiatric Clinics of North America, 15,* 759–777.

Christ, G. (2000). *Healing children's grief: Surviving a parent's death from cancer.* New York, NY: Oxford University Press.

Contro, N., Larson, J., Scofield S., Sourkes, B., & Cohen, H. (2002). Family perspectives on the quality of pediatric palliative care. *Archives of Pediatric & Adolescent Medicine, 156,* 14–19.

Contro, N., Larson, J., Scofield S., Sourkes, B., & Cohen, H. (2004). Hospital staff and family perspectives regarding quality of pediatric palliative care. *Pediatrics, 114,* 1248–1252.

Cooley, W. C. (2001). Family-centered care in pediatric practice. In R. A. Hoekelman (Ed.), *Primary pediatric care* (pp. 712–714). St. Louis, MO: Mosby.

Csikai, E. L., & Chaitin, E. (2006). *Ethics in end-of-life decisions in social work practice.* Chicago, IL: Lyceum Press.

Curtis, J. R., Engelberg, R. A., Wenrich, M. D., Shannon, S. E., Treece, P. D., & Rubenfeld, G. D. (2005). Missed opportunities during family conferences about end-of-life care in the ICU. *American Journal of Respiratory Critical Care Medicine, 171,* 844–849.

Curtis, J. R., & Rubenfeld, G. D. (2005). Improving palliative care for patients in the intensive care unit. *Journal of Palliative Medicine, 8,* 840–854.

Curtis, J. R., & White, D. B. (2008). Practical guidance for evidence-based ICU family conferences. *Chest, 134,* 835–843.

Davidson, J. E., Powers, K., Hedayat, K. M., Tieszen, M., Kon, A. A., Shepard, E., ... American College of Critical Care Medicine Task Force 2004–2005, Society of Critical Care Medicine. (2007). Clinical practice guidelines for support of the family in the patient-centered intensive care unit: American College of Critical Care Medicine Task Force 2004–2005. *Critical Care Medicine, 35,* 605–622.

Davies, B., & Connaughty, S. (2002). Pediatric end-of-life care: Lessons learned from parents. *Journal of Nursing Administration, 32,* 5–6.

Feudtner, C., Kang, T. I., Hexem, K. R., Friedrichsdorf, S. J., Osenga, K., Siden, H., ... Wolfe, J. (2011). Pediatric palliative care patients: A prospective multicenter cohort study. *Pediatrics, 127,* 1094–1101.

Field, M. J., & Behrman, R. E. (Eds.). (2003). *When children die: Improving palliative and end-of-life care for children and their families.* Washington, DC: National Academy Press.

Fine, E., Reid, M. C., Shengelia, R., & Adelman, R. D. (2010). Directly observed patient–physician discussions in palliative and end-of-life care: A systematic review of the literature. *Journal of Palliative Medicine, 13,* 595–603.

Fineberg, I. C. (2010). Social work perspectives on family communication and family conferences in palliative care. *Progress in Palliative Care, 18*(4), 213–220.

Fineberg, I. C., Kawashima, M., & Asch, S. M. (2011). Communication with families facing life-threatening illness: A research-based model for family conferences. *Journal of Palliative Medicine, 14,* 421–427.

Frazier A., Frazier, H., & Warren, N. A. (2009). A discussion of family-centered care within the pediatric intensive care unit. *Critical Care Nursing Quarterly, 33,* 82–86.

Friebert, S. (2009). *NHPCO facts and figures: Pediatric palliative and hospice care in America*. Alexandria, VA: National Hospice and Palliative Care Organization.

Friedman, D. L., Hilden, J. N., & Powaski, K. (2005). Issues and challenges in palliative care for children with cancer. *Current Pain and Headache Reports, 9*, 249–255.

Gries, C. J., Engelberg, R. A., Kross, E. K., Zatzick, D., Nielsen, E. L., Downey, L., & Curtis, J. R. (2010). Predictors of symptoms of post–traumatic stress and depression in family members after patient death in the intensive care unit. *Chest, 137*, 280–287.

Hays, R. M., Valentine, J., Haynes, G., Geyer, J. R., Villareale, N., McKinistry, B., … Churchill, S. S. (2006). The Seattle Pediatric Palliative Care Project: Effects on family satisfaction and health-related quality of life. *Journal of Palliative Medicine, 9*, 716–728.

Heyland, D. K., Cook, D. J., Rocker, G. M., Dodek, P. M., Kutsogiannis, D. J., Peters, S., … O'Callaghan, C. J. (2003). Decision-making in the ICU: Perspectives of the substitute decision-maker. *Intensive Care Medicine, 29*, 75–82.

Hinds, P. S., Schum, L., Baker, J. N., & Wolfe, J. (2005). Key factors affecting dying children and their families. *Journal of Palliative Medicine, 8*(Suppl. 1), 70–78.

Hooyman, N. R., & Kramer, B. J. (2006). *Living through loss: Interventions across the life span*. New York, NY: Columbia University Press.

Hutton, N. (2002). Pediatric palliative care: The time has come. *Archives of Pediatric and Adolescent Medicine, 156*, 9–10.

Johnson, B. H. (2000). Family-centered care: Four decades of progress. *Families, Systems, & Health, 18*, 133–156.

Johnson, B. H., & Eichner, J. M. (2003). Family-centered care and the pediatrician's role. *Pediatrics, 112*, 691–696.

Jones, B. L., Parker-Raley, J., Higgerson, R., Christie, L. M., Legett, S., & Greathouse, J. (2008). Finding the right words: The use of Allow Natural Death (AND) and DNR in pediatric palliative care. *Journal for Healthcare Quality, 30*(5), 55–63.

Jones, B. L., Sampson, M., Greathouse, J., Legett, S., Higgerson, R. A., & Christie, L. (2007). Comfort and confidence levels of health care professionals providing pediatric palliative care in the intensive care unit. *Journal of Social Work in End-of-Life and Palliative Care, 3*, 39–58.

Jonsen, A. R., Siegler, M., & Winslade, W. J. (2002). *Clinical ethics: A practical approach to ethical decisions in clinical medicine* (5th ed.). New York, NY: McGraw-Hill.

Kreicbergs, U. C., Lannen, P., Onelov, E., & Wolfe, J. (2007). Parental grief after losing a child to cancer: Impact of professional and social support on long-term outcomes. *Journal of Clinical Oncology, 25*, 3307–3312.

Lannen, P. K., Wolfe, J., Prigerson, H. G., Onelov, E., & Kreicbergs, U. C. (2008). Unresolved grief in a national sample of bereaved parents: Impaired mental and physical health 4 to 9 years later. *Journal of Clinical Oncology, 26*, 5870–5876.

Lautrette, A., Darmon, M., Megarbane, B., Joly, L. M., Chevret, S., Adrie, C., … Azoulay, E. (2007). A communication strategy and brochure for relatives of patients dying in the ICU. *New England Journal of Medicine, 356*, 469–478.

Mack, J. W., Hilden, J. M., Watterson, J., Moore, C., Turner, B., Grier, H. E., … Wolfe, J. (2005). Parent and physician perspectives on quality of care at the end of life in children with cancer. *Journal of Clinical Oncology, 23*, 9155–9161.

MacLachlan, M. (2007). *Culture and health* (2nd ed.). Hoboken, NJ: Wiley & Sons.

Martin, J. A., Kung, H. C., Mathews, T. J., Hovert D. L., Strobino D. M., Guyer, B., & Sutton, S. R. (2008). Annual summary of vital statistics: 2006. *Pediatrics, 121,* 788–801.

McDonagh, J. R., Elliott, T. B., Engelberg, R. A., Treece, P. D., Shannon, S. E., Rubenfeld, G. D., ... Curtis, J. R. (2004). Family satisfaction with family conferences about end-of-life care in the ICU: Increased proportion of family speech is associated with increased satisfaction. *Critical Care Medicine, 32,* 1484–1488.

Meert, K., Briller, S. H., Thurston, C., & Schim, S. M. (2008). Exploring parents' environmental needs at the time of a child's death in the pediatric intensive care unit. *Pediatric Critical Care Medicine, 9,* 623–628.

Meert, K. L., Donaldson A. E., Newth, C. J., Harrison, R., Berger, J., Zimmerman, J., ... Eunice Kennedy Shriver National Institute of Child Health and Human Development Collaborative Pediatric Critical Care Research Network. (2010). Complicated grief and associated risk factors among parents following a child's death in the pediatric intensive care unit. *Archives of Pediatrics & Adolescent Medicine, 164,* 1045–1051.

Meert, K. L., Thurston, C. S., & Thomas, R. (2001). Parental coping and bereavement outcome after the death of a child in the pediatric intensive care unit. *Pediatric Critical Care Medicine, 2,* 324–328.

Meier, D. E., & Beresford, L. (2008). Social workers advocate for a seat at palliative care table. *Journal of Palliative Medicine, 11,* 10–14.

Melnyk, B. M., Feinstein, N., & Fairbanks, E. (2006). Two decades of evidence to support implementation of the COPE program as standard practice with parents of young unexpectedly hospitalized/critically ill children and premature infants. *Pediatric Nursing, 32,* 475–481.

Meyer, E. C., Burns, J. P., Griffith, J. L., & Truog, R. D. (2002). Parental perspectives on end-of-life care in the pediatric intensive care unit. *Critical Care Medicine, 30,* 226–231.

Meyer, E. C., Ritholz, M. D., Burns, J. P., & Truog, R. D. (2006). Improving the quality of end-of-life care in the pediatric intensive care unit: Parents' priorities and recommendations. *Pediatrics, 117,* 649–657.

National Association of Children's Hospitals and Related Institutions. (2009). Retrieved from http://www.childrenshospitals.net

Pochard, F., Azoulay, E., Chevret, S., Lemaire, F., Hubert, P., Canoui, P., ... French FAMIREA Group. (2001). Symptoms of anxiety and depression in family members of intensive care unit patients: Ethical hypothesis regarding decision-making capacity. *Critical Care Medicine, 29,* 1893–1897.

Rait, D., & Lederberg, M. (1989). The family of the cancer patient. In J. C. Holland, & J. H. Rowland (Eds.), *Handbook of psychooncology: Psychological care of the patient with cancer* (pp. 555–601). New York, NY: Oxford University Press.

Raymer, M., & Reese, D. (2004). The history of social work in hospice. In J. Berzoff, & P. Silverman (Eds.), *Living with dying: A handbook for end-of-life practitioners* (pp. 150–160). New York, NY: Columbia University Press.

Sahler, O. J. (2000). The child and death. *Pediatric Review, 21,* 350–353.

Sands, R., Manning, J. C., Vyas, H., & Rashid, A. (2009) Characteristics of deaths in paediatric intensive care: A 10-year study. *Nursing in Critical Care, 14,* 235–240.

Schneiderman, L. J., Gilmer, T., Teetzel, H. D., Dugan, D. O., Blustein, J., Cranford, R., … Young, E. W. (2003). Effect of ethics consultations on nonbeneficial life-sustaining treatments in the intensive care setting: A randomized controlled trial. *Journal of the American Medical Association, 290*, 1166–1172.

Selph, R. B., Shiang, J., Engelberg, R., Curtis, J. R., & White, D. B. (2008). Empathy and life support decisions in intensive care units. *Journal of General Internal Medicine, 23*, 1311–1317.

Shudy, M., de Almeida M. L., Ly, S., Landon, C., Groft, S., Jenkins, T. L., & Nicholson, C. E. (2006). Impact of pediatric critical illness and injury on families: A systematic literature review. *Pediatrics, 118*(Suppl. 3), S203–S218.

Smith, A. B., Hefley, G. C., & Anand, K. J. (2007). Parent bed spaces in the PICU: Effect on parental stress. *Pediatric Nursing, 33*, 215–221.

Stapleton, R. D., Engelberg, R. A., Wenrich, M. D., Goss, C. H., & Curtis, J. R. (2006). Clinician statements and family satisfaction with family conferences in the intensive care unit. *Critical Care Medicine, 34*, 1679–1685.

Studdert, D. M., Mello, M. M., Burns, J. P., Puopolo, A. A., Galper, B. Z., Truog, R. D., & Brennan, T. A. (2003). Conflict in the care of patients with prolonged stay in the ICU: Types, sources, and predictors. *Intensive Care Medicine, 29*, 1489–1497.

Teno, J. M., Clarridge, B. R., Casey, V. A., Welch, L. C., Wetle, T., Shield, R., & Mor, V. (2004). Family perspectives on end-of-life care at the last place of care. *Journal of the American Medical Association, 291*, 88–93.

Truog, R. D., Meyer, E. C., & Burns, J. P. (2006). Toward interventions to improve end-of-life care in the pediatric intensive care unit. *Critical Care Medicine, 34*(Suppl. 11), S373–S379.

Tulsky J. A. (2005). Interventions to enhance communication among patients, providers, and families. *Journal of Palliative Medicine, 8*(Suppl. 1), S95–S102.

Weissman, D. E., Quill, T. E., & Arnold, R. M. (2010a). The family meeting: End-of-life goal setting and future planning. *Journal of Palliative Medicine, 13*, 462–463.

Weissman, D. E., Quill, T. E., & Arnold, R. M. (2010b). Helping surrogates make decisions. *Journal of Palliative Medicine, 13*, 461–462.

West, H. F., Engelberg, R. A., Wenrich, M. D., & Curtis, J. R. (2005). Expressions of nonabandonment during the intensive care unit family conference. *Journal of Palliative Medicine, 8*, 797–807.

White, D. B., Malvar, G., Karr, J., Lo, B., & Curtis, J. R. (2010). Expanding the paradigm of the physician's role in surrogate decision making: An empirically derived framework. *Critical Care Medicine, 38*, 743–750.

World Health Organization. (2010). *Palliative care.* Retrieved from http://www.who.int/cancer/palliative/en

Bereaved Parents' Perspectives on Pediatric Palliative Care

RHONDA ROBERT

*Division of Pediatrics, The University of Texas MD Anderson Cancer
Center Children's Cancer Hospital, Houston, Texas, USA*

DONNA S. ZHUKOVSKY

*Division of Pediatrics, The University of Texas MD Anderson Cancer
Center Children's Cancer Hospital, Houston, Texas, USA, and Department
of Palliative Care and Rehabilitation Medicine, The University of Texas MD
Anderson Cancer Center, Houston, Texas, USA*

RIZA MAURICIO

*Division of Pediatrics, The University of Texas MD Anderson Cancer
Center Children's Cancer Hospital, Houston, Texas, USA*

KATHERINE GILMORE

*Department of Symptom Research, The University of Texas MD
Anderson Cancer Center, Houston, Texas, USA*

SHIRLEY MORRISON

*Department of Nursing, Texas Women's University HoustonCenter,
Houston, Texas*

GUADALUPE R. PALOS

*Office of Cancer Survivorship, The University of Texas MD Anderson
Cancer Center, Houston, Texas, USA*

This study's goal was to describe and begin to understand the experience of bereaved parents whose deceased child had received pediatric oncology services at a tertiary comprehensive cancer center.

The authors would like to thank the MD Anderson Cancer Center Children's Art Project™ whose financial support made this study possible and the children, parents, and clinicians who gave so generously of themselves to help other children and their families achieve a better quality of life.

Focus groups were conducted with parents whose children were age 10 years and older at the time of death. Potential participants were contacted by mail and telephone. Sessions were audiotaped and transcribed verbatim. The ATLAS.ti qualitative software program was used to identify and analyze dominant themes. Fourteen parents identified four major themes: standards of care, emotional care, communication, and social support. Bereaved parents discussed the challenges associated with institutional procedures and interpersonal aspects of care in anticipation of and following their child's death. The results of these personal narratives may be used to guide care plans and deliver pediatric palliative and end-of-life interventions.

INTRODUCTION

Pediatric palliative care (PPC) must be an integral component of both cancer care and social work practice (Altilio, Gardia, & Otis-Green, 2007; Altilio & Otis-Green, 2005; Gwyther et al., 2005). The growing number of PPC reports, standards of care, and programs aim to improve patient and family quality of life. All of the above emphasize the importance of an integrated interdisciplinary model of care (Foster, Lafond, Reggio, & Hinds, 2010). The Institute of Medicine report (2003b) "When Children Die" identified the need for development of appropriate palliative care and core values in the provision of pediatric-specific palliation. As a result of these efforts, social workers with knowledge, skills, and experience in PPC are increasingly in demand (Orloff, 2011; Jones & Phillips, 2011). Several professional organizations such as the Social Work in Hospice and Palliative Care Network (SWHPN), National Association of Social Workers (NASW), Association of Oncology Social Workers (AOSW), and the National Quality Forum (NQF) have developed national agendas, networks, and strategies to support the profession's evolution and need for expertise in palliative care (Altilio, Otis-Green, & Dahlin, 2008; Bern-Klug, Kramer, & Linder, 2005; Altilio et al., 2007; Christ & Blacker, 2006).

The NASW (2004) supported this movement by developing best practice guidelines and core competencies for social workers in the *Standards and Social Work Practice in Palliative and End-of-Life Care* (Table 1). To further support the competencies unique to this specialty, the Association of Pediatric Oncology Social Workers (APOSW, 2005) identified six core elements distinct to palliative care: (a) providing specialized PPC service; (b) being an advocate and educator; (c) providing supportive counseling for the

TABLE 1 NASW Standards and Social Work Practice in Palliative and End-of-Life Care

1. Ethics and values
2. Knowledge
3. Assessment
4. Intervention/treatment planning
5. Attitude/self-awareness
6. Empowerment and advocacy
7. Documentation
8. Interdisciplinary teamwork
9. Cultural competence
10. Continuing education
11. Supervision, leadership, and training

Source: National Association of Social Workers Standards, available at http://www.socialworkers.org/practice/bereavement/standards/default.asp

child, sibling, and parents; (d) listening to fears, hopes, and concerns; (e) conducting psychosocial assessments based on the child and family; and (f) counseling the family in grief and bereavement.

To date, delivery of services and models of social work practice in PPC have been primarily guided by clinical practices, experience, and ethics. Evidence-based practice that combines well-researched interventions with the PPC social work practice has been limited, particularly examining bereaved parents' mourning process regarding the loss of their child (Kramer, Christ, Bern-Klug, & Francoeur, 2005; Palos, 2011).

Patients, parents, and other family members who have utilized oncology care services for children who have died of their disease or its complications are experts regarding optimal palliative care. In most cases, after a child dies, opportunities for parents or other family members to provide feedback on the care received by their child are limited or nonexistent. In this qualitative study, the investigators sought to understand the needs and experiences of bereaved parents whose child had received care at one National Cancer Institute-designated comprehensive cancer center. The investigators were particularly interested in the parents' perceptions of the care received by their child, their expectations of palliative care, and recommendations on how best to improve palliative care for children with cancer and their parents.

METHODS

Focus group methodology was believed to be ideal for gathering information and minimizing the potential for participant distress. Group meetings are a familiar format and tend to be associated with relaxed, spontaneous discussions and hence, nonthreatening. An ice-breaker question was posed to open the discussion, set participants at ease, and encourage a common bond amongst participants. Participants were encouraged to express their points freely and in their own terms. Nonverbal communication was utilized to convey support and understanding. The facilitator fostered an exchange of information through query. Emotional information was acknowledged, validated, and balanced with moving the session forward once participants were ready. Participants, given the shared experience of a child's death, provided mutual support. Direct observation and face-to-face interactions between participants and investigators allowed for ongoing assessment of participant's emotional status during study participation and, if needed, timely access to support.

Study Sample and Procedures

Eligible focus group participants were parents of children who had been treated at a tertiary comprehensive cancer center and were at least 10 years old at the time of death. The child's age limit was intended to balance sampling variability and homogeneity (Mayan, 2001). Older children have a greater capacity for communicating their internal experiences and needs. Consequently, parents were able to have more information from their children while they were providing care through the illness. The sample included parents whose child died a minimum of 1 year prior to the study. The criterion regarding time since death was established to minimize parents' distress during study participation. Parents whose child had died prior to May 2007 met this particular eligibility criterion, as enrollment screening began in May 2008. To minimize the burden of participation, only parents residing within the state where the center is located were eligible. A potential participant was excluded if cognitive impairment, developmental delay, or emotional status would have limited participation in a group discussion, as determined by the clinical investigators. Parents were recruited for three focus group sessions. Institutional Review Board approval was obtained to for the procedures and implementation of the study.

The focus groups were held between May 2008 and June 2009. Parents of 47 children were eligible to participate. Contact was successful with 25 families. Of those 25 families, 9 declined and 7 expressed possible interest at a later date. Reasons given for declining participation were logistical barriers ($n = 4$) and anticipated emotional distress ($n = 2$); one family politely declined without giving a reason, and two families committed but neither attended nor cancelled. Three parents declined focus group participation but provided immediate feedback during the recruitment telephone call and requested to have their comments considered. Of the 25 families who did respond to contact attempts, 14 parents from 9 families (36%) agreed to participate in the study. Three focus groups were conducted, with two, seven, and five parents in the first, second, and third focus groups, respectively.

Potential participants received a letter containing an invitation to participate in the study, a brief explanation of the study, and instructions on how to contact the investigators for further information. A stamped, addressed return postcard was included, and recipients were asked to indicate interest in learning more about participation or to decline further contact regarding the study. Parents who indicated interest were telephoned to discuss their availability to attend focus group sessions. A treatment provider well known to the parents placed the follow-up telephone call to those who did not return the postcard after 2 weeks.

Travel reimbursement (parking and fuel expenses) and a $25.00 gift card were given as a way to acknowledge the parents' effort and investment in participation. Parents were encouraged to attend with another caregiver. The recruitment procedures did not allow for random sampling but rather criterion sampling, in which individuals who had experienced the phenomenon of interest were selected (Creswell, 2006).

Confirmation telephone calls were placed shortly before the date of each focus group session. Written informed consent was obtained at the focus group site. Ample opportunity was provided for questions to be asked and answered before the meeting was initiated.

Procedures and Measures

Exploratory group interview methods were used during the focus group sessions (Morgan, 1993). The study investigators—including a palliative care physician (DSZ), a pediatric psychologist (RR), and a social worker with expertise in focus group research (GRP)—served as content experts in developing an interview script. Content domains were derived from a literature review. This draft was reviewed by an internationally recognized expert in PPC and focus group methodology (P. Hinds, personal communication, 2007). The script was edited in accordance with the feedback.

Following well-established qualitative focus group methods (Creswell, 2006; Miles, 1994), GRP trained the other investigators to record detailed field notes and behavioral observations during the sessions. In the focus group session, bereaved parents were invited to reflect on and discuss their experience of palliative care during their child's illness. Following an introductory explanation, sequences of open-ended, semi-structured questions were posed by the facilitator (GRP) that addressed the topics of communication, emotional care, treatment decision making, spiritual care, and symptom management. The following is a sample interview statement: "As your child's death was approaching, our goal was to help as best as possible. We would like to know what went well during that time and what did not go well."

The discussions were audiotaped and transcribed by a professional transcriptionist.

To optimize confidentiality, personal identifiers were omitted from the transcriptions and the data were secured both physically and electronically. In addition to clinical data regarding the deceased child's diagnosis, demographic data on the parent(s) and the child were collected.

Data Analysis

Demographic data were analyzed descriptively. The group discussions were transcribed verbatim and provided the basis for the content analysis. ATLAS. ti, Version 4 (ATLAS.ti Scientific Software Development GmbH, Berlin, Germany) was used to organize and analyze qualitative data. A six-member research team (three investigators, two advanced practice nurses, and one research coordinator) participated in an exploratory analysis of the textual content to identify codes for all three focus group transcripts. Major themes evolved by grouping textual codes similar in content together. Disagreements over themes were resolved by consensus. Original statements were selected as examples to justify the categories created. The field notes were reviewed during the data analysis and observations of participants' nonverbal behaviors were added to provide rich descriptions of the phenomenon being explored.

Methodological Challenges and Working Solutions

Initial contact and recruitment methods resulted in too few study participants. The study investigators sought advice from the institution's Pediatric Supportive Care Committee's parent advisors. The parent advisors had particular interest in improving palliative care services and programs and volunteered to assist. They re-worded the recruitment letter and explained to the investigators the importance of a familiar treatment provider contacting the parent. The parent advisors emphasized the importance of a person-to-person connection as opposed to an impersonal mailed letter. Some of the parents advisors explained that they had reflexively thrown away institutional mailings after their child had died and suggested this might be one reason for the low response rate.

 The parents who expressed interest in study participation had several requests that had not been anticipated or accounted for in the eligibility criteria. During the recruitment phone call, parents asked to participate by telephone, speak in a first or native language with the assistance of an interpreter (despite being fluent in English), and attend a focus group with the support of a spouse. The eligibility criteria and recruitment methods were reworked accordingly.

RESULTS

Focus Group Participants

The mean age ($\pm SD$) of the focus group participants was 51 years (± 6). Mothers and fathers were equally represented. Their children had been, on average, 15 years of age (± 3) at the time of their deaths. Six of the children were boys and three were girls. The cancer types were central nervous system malignancy ($N=1$), leukemia ($N=3$), or solid tumor ($N=5$). All participants were married and their spouses (husband or wife) either shared equally in parenting responsibilities or had had consistent contact but less than half of the parenting responsibilities. Ten participants were White, three were Mexican American, and one was Arab American. Educational background varied from some high school to advanced degrees. All were employed full time except for two homemakers. All but one had living children (sibling to the deceased patient; see Table 2).

Focus Group Themes

Of the five content areas identified during literature review for the interview script development, emotional care and communication generated the most discussion. The number of related comments for these two themes was 5 to 6 times than the number of comments regarding the content areas of decision making, spiritual care, or symptom management. The latter three topics generated minimal yet pertinent discussion. Informed, collaborative, step-wise

TABLE 2 Demographic and Clinical Characteristics of Bereaved Parents and Deceased Children

Bereaved parents ($N = 14$)	
Mean age (years $\pm SD$)	51 ± 5.8
Gender (male:female)	7:7
Ethnicity (N)	
Hispanic	3
Non-Hispanic White	10
Other	1
Educational level (N)	
Some high school	2
High school graduate	1
Associate degree/some college	4
Bachelor's degree	3
Graduate degree	4
Employment status (N)	
Full-time outside the home	12
Homemaker	2
Deceased children ($N = 9$)	
Mean age at diagnosis (years $\pm SD$)	14.9 ± 3.1
Mean age at relapse (years $\pm SD$)	17.0 ± 2.0
Gender (male:female)	6:3
Ethnicity (N)	
Hispanic	1
Non-Hispanic White	7
Other	1
Cancer diagnosis (N)	
Leukemia	3
Glioblastoma multiforme	1
Other solid tumor	5

decision making had been desired as opposed to abrupt, unilateral decision making. Parents welcomed spiritual care and symptom management before a critical event presented, as opposed to a reactionary offering during an event.

Two unexpected themes emerged during the focus groups: standards of care and social support. The standards of care theme received more comments than any of the five content areas identified in the literature review. The dominant themes and corresponding sample narratives are discussed below, beginning with the most dominant theme: standards of care, emotional care, communication, and social support.

STANDARDS OF CARE

The phrase *standards of care* was intended to capture basic aspects of patient care and was not limited to palliative or end-of-life care. Basic aspects of care and their importance during this critical period of illness were highlighted in the focus group discussions. Themes that emerged from further analysis of standards of care included: (a) knowledge of processes and negotiation within the institution; (b) development of trusted relationships with treatment providers; (c) personalized patient accommodation; and (d) accommodation for caregivers and visitors, including young children. Table 3 shows verbatim quotations from participants, and Table 4 lists clinical practices suggested by the participant quotations.

Comments regarding *knowledge of processes and negotiation within the institution* pertained to the initial phase of a treatment. Identification and selection of the optimal clinic and primary treatment team is ideally determined by both the age-appropriateness of the treatment setting and the expertise of the individual providers. Parents did not have the experience necessary to identify clinics and treatment teams as choices: "The adult unit should have never been an option. If the pediatric unit could handle what [our child] had, … that's where we should have went." Both the degree to which the treatment setting was age appropriate and the expertise of the individual providers were valued. The participants described the characteristics of clinics, environments, and programs for adult patients to be "ill-fitting" for pediatric, adolescent, and young adult patients. Provider expertise was important, but in hindsight the participants found that the expertise was attainable in both the adult and pediatric settings.

Understanding the treatment team's organization and the providers' specialized roles was more complex than anticipated. At the beginning of treatment, the concept of having the involvement of many doctors versus one doctor had been mystifying: "After the 5th or 6th week, I figured out, 'Hey, I've got a dozen doctors, not one. No one comes right out and tells you.'" Parents suggested that meeting consultants and allied service providers earlier in the course of illness and treatment would have been helpful: "From the beginning, give all the resources, so it's not slipped in at the end."

TABLE 3 Theme: Standards of Care

Knowledge of processes and negotiation within the system
- The adult unit should have never been an option. If the pediatric unit could handle what [our child] had, … that's where we should have went.
- After the 5th or 6th week, I figured out, "Hey, I've got a dozen doctors, not one." No one comes right out and tells you.
- From the beginning, give all the resources, so it's not slipped in at the end.

Development of trusted relationships
- If somebody wasn't there throughout the whole ordeal, I wasn't interested in talking to them … . It's pretty hard to open up with somebody you don't know at that point in time in your life … . I go back to the relationship and the trust.
- The same person drawing blood every time [was helpful].
- A different person every single time drew his blood … . Sometimes he had to be stuck 2–3 times because they didn't ask for the right tests … . [My son] said, "Dad, that lady was so good. I didn't even feel the needle." I said, "We'll just ask for her every time." He said, "No. I don't want to offend the other one" … . The lady that tried to draw blood 6 times before giving up.
- Continuity was not there. Our doctor transferred out in the middle.
- I would have liked the same doctor the whole time … . The biggest shock [came when] our doctor said, "I've been here 9 months." That's not what I wanted to hear. I [wanted someone who had] treated thousands.
- [We needed an] integrated [medical] team.
- [Our daughter] had a medication reaction, and she was going into cardiac arrest; and then we were in for the next chemo; and they tried to give her the same medicine … . If I hadn't been there they would have given it to her again.
- [Staff should] respect [that] people inside the rooms are facing death … are … in pain, while someone else is laughing [in a] loud voice. It hurts.
- The [inpatient nurses] were wonderful, but ran … from one patient to the next, … going 90 miles an hour, trying to keep up. [In ICU], … you got a lot of special attention and that meant the world to us. The nurse could just sit there to make him comfortable, even though we were there … . That meant the most to us at that point in time—to have a lot of support right there, compassionate people.
- Near the end of his life, [my son] was in pain. The doctor came with a student, and asked, "When do you think we should give him this amount or the other?" I was very disappointed. You have to consider that this child is in pain. If you want to ask this question [of the student], get out. It should be you and a doctor.
- [The] nurse was horrible, really bad, no love, no caring, no bedside manner. It was, "This is the way it is, period. Don't ask any more questions." She chewed me out one time … just unloaded on us … didn't have any patience.
- In the ICU, people were supposed to be gloved and masked. [But they weren't]. I came unwound! [Our daughter] said [to the staff], "You are supposed to have glove and mask on." This made me feel insecure.
- At the funeral, the first two people who showed up were [hospital staff]. They came early and were thereafter. They grow to love these kids. They're not just patients.

Personalized patient accommodation
- They'd … immediately put him in a room, … in a bed, comfortable, watching TV … . It hurt for him to sit.
- The less rules, the better. What was perfect for [one patient] was totally different for [our son]…. Ask the kid.
- [The staff said,] "We'll have his wheelchair in about 4 months." I said, "He's gonna [sic] be gone in 4 months." They said, "Well, I'm sorry. That's the best we can do."

Accommodation of caregivers and visitors, including young children
- Always have a bed [for parents] to sleep on instead of those chairs.
- We always liked to be with our child regardless [which ICU rules did not allow].
- We had to stand. [The ICU] didn't have chairs.

(Continued)

TABLE 3 *Continued*

- [In the ICU, parents had to go elsewhere to bathe].
- ICU was horrible. Sitting there waiting and waiting [to return to my child's room. Staff sent me out and] didn't come back to get me.
- We were locked up here during [a hurricane]. They had food for [the patient] but not for [the family].
- I got a call looking for an oxygen payment—after she had died. I'm pretty sure we didn't use that oxygen…. We had to send a death certificate.
- We had the whole waiting room…. [Staff] never said a word. They just let us be there to take care of him.
- The ICU nurses were angry that nobody was taking care of [the patient's young sibling]. [People far away from home] need support.

In addition, participants felt overlooked because they were not informed about specialized services or programs earlier in treatment. Participants related that as the child neared death, they were less inclined to accept a newly initiated service or relate to a new provider. Intimacy was highly valued at the child's end of life. Trusted others were increasingly relied upon, and parents limited their child's interactions to persons well known to the family. Parents valued *trusting relationships with providers*. Care was considered optimal when the provider and patient had grown to know one another: "At the funeral, the first two people who showed up were [hospital staff]. They came early and were thereafter. They grow to love these kids. They're

TABLE 4 Suggested Standard of Care Tenets

- Treat youth in a youth-oriented environment
- Develop relationships with patients: be well-known, trusted, and available
- Minimize wait time, maximize comfort
- Be flexible and accommodating: persons first, rules second
- Minimize needle sticks and blood draws
- Be consistent—e.g., with use of gloves and masks
- Identify needs and find solutions
- Work together
- Say goodbye
- Implement institutional billing delays to allow parents time to grieve
- Anticipate information needed and provide the information in a concise manner
- Support togetherness—e.g., avoid enforced parent-child separation
- Accommodate siblings
- During hospitalization
  - Provide parents a chair, bed, bath, and food
  - Provide teaching opportunities away from the bedside
  - Assume someone is grieving and create a calm, peaceful setting
- Help patients/parents/families determine when it is time to transition from curative to palliative goals
  - Discuss treatment setting options
  - Offer prognostic news as related medical information presents
  - Be candid but sensitive when informing families there is no cure for their child and when their child is approaching the end of life

not just patients." Regardless of the task at hand, whether a blood draw or medication decision, trust and familiarity between providers, patients, and parents bred confidence, security, a sense of what to expect, matching of expectations, and overall strong relationships. Time, interest, care, sensitivity, empathy, consideration, and love from the treatment provider was highly valued. Across the three focus groups, parents strongly agreed that working with the same provider and team was a key factor in building trust, relationships, and communication.

Personalized accommodation, meaning individualized care in which persons' emotional and physical needs take priority to institutional policies, rules, and norms. Parents believed that every child was unique, as was their diagnosis, and both required creative and personalized solutions and a dynamic work environment: "The less rules, the better. What was perfect for [one patient] was totally different for [our son] … . Ask the kid." *Personalized accommodation* extended beyond the patient and included caregivers and visitors. Of primary importance was that these parents wanted to be with their children and enforced parent-child separations had been disturbing. During their child's hospitalization, parents needed access to a shower, food, and seating, as well as a bed for the night. Visitors, including young children, were essential sources of support and their visits were valued. After the child's death, parents needed emotional accommodation in the form of special dispensation from hospital-related bills and payment time lines. Parents felt barraged by hospital-related bills received proximal to the child's death: "I got a call looking for an oxygen payment—after she had died. I'm pretty sure we didn't use that oxygen … . We had to send a death certificate." Parents shared that they decompressed emotionally by focusing on funeral-related events and expenses rather than confronting the hospital bills.

EMOTIONAL CARE

The topic of *emotional care*, both before and after the child's death, generated extensive discussion. Comments on this topic are located in Table 5. Parents described the child's ambivalence to talk about death and the importance of the child having control regarding end-of-life discussions: "Our daughter wanted to talk about [terminal cancer], then didn't … . [A doctor asked her], 'What are you afraid of? … Dying? … Why?' … That made it easier for her to talk to us, … to be in control … . She could plan her funeral." The participants also described the importance of providers' skill in talking about death. Parents believed that some providers had avoided talking about death or relied on a set method or technique for having an end-of-life discussion. Both avoidance and rote methods for talking about death were troubling. Parents suggested the importance of tailoring end-of-life discussions according to the needs of those participating.

TABLE 5 Theme: Emotional Care

Patient

- Our daughter wanted to talk about [terminal cancer], then didn't … . [A doctor asked her], "What are you afraid of? … Dying? … Why?" … That made it easier for her to talk to us, … to be in control … . She could plan her funeral.
- It's keeping control.
- [The psychologist] was very supportive of him and of us. They were wonderful … in child life, the pastors, … all the nurses made us comfortable. Communication was good.
- Let kids have control, even at 5 or 6 [years of age]. You have to know which doctors aren't good with having the conversation because the palliative care [doctor can then] step up and have that conversation.
- I know that in palliative care, they take care of the pain, constipation, all sorts of cushioning the end-of- life … . [My son] did not want to see them … . He knows that the palliative care is close to death. I think the word was a little strong for him … . He [searched] the Internet to find out what he wanted. He didn't want to talk about … the end of his life.
- We didn't have the cure. [Death was] not what I wanted to discuss. … When a doctor tells him, "We don't have a cure," tell me that. Don't tell him that. I am here for him—it was too much for him to deal with. One time he told me, "Mom, I'm really worried [others] are giving me a death sentence." They should not tell him everything. I know my son. He was telling them, "Tell me everything," but you shouldn't. I see the consequences of someone telling him that he will die. It's really hard … . There is hope, miracles, positive thinking. We never know what will happen … . You see in everyone's faces that it's the end. You should deal with him as he is going to live, we never know … . In the end I was like a policeman. I didn't want anybody to tell my child that he is going to die. If you have something positive, you can tell him, but if you don't, please just get out.
- We loved, bonded with [our son's doctor]. [A school] rule is, "If you don't go to school that day you can't participate in activities or sports that night." [The doctor] said, "There are loopholes, ways around it. I'll be right back." He [returned with a] letter, which basically prescribed the football game.
- When the time comes, do you want your child to be in the conversation? No matter how hard it is, everybody wants the truth, but I don't think covering it over and over and over is helpful. Be sensitive. Trust comes from time and relationship. It was difficult when doctors that I have never seen come in at the end. [They weren't going to] make his life more comfortable. They were researching, and we were trying to participate, but once we crossed that line, it was time for us, not them.
- As far as end-of-life issues, when it comes to teens, it's not a subject they want to discuss.
- We were about quality of life, and every day, regardless of what was going on, chemo, puking our guts up, whatever it might have been, we were laughing and smiling 10 or 15 minutes later. That's how we dealt with it. You have bad days but then you have good ones.

Parent as caregiver

- When [my husband] showed up and they talked about DNR, he didn't understand. [The doctor] explained it again, I couldn't. My husband needed the medical guy to say it. For them to take that time, to know today, in the eyes of the parents, we are your only patient. That made it bearable.
- At that point in time [end-of-life] … I wouldn't be willing to open up to somebody I didn't know.
- I "what if" myself every day.
- Postdeath, [parents need an] awareness of what to expect, the shades of normal, and how to handle the [deceased's] room and siblings.

TABLE 5 *Continued*

Parent as spouse
• My husband and I are different. He is not participating in this focus group because he won't come here again. When [our daughter] got sick, I was here all the time. He couldn't do it psychologically, emotionally.
• What do you do when one spouse wants to pack up the stuff and the other can't?
Siblings
• Our daughter was ... in college, but in hindsight it probably would have been good for someone to talk to her.
• Right before [our son] died, [our daughter was] ... vandalizing school, ... throwing mud, ... piercing her own ears, like self-mutilation.
• It's really hard for her because he's not here, so she hasn't dealt with the daily grief.
• I think she's got a lot of grieving still to do. I think she's ignored it and avoided it, but she hasn't been home.
• Our son is 25 and still wrestling with it.
• Our son is 19, and we as parents can't fix them except to love them.
• It's been the worst since she has been gone. We've been in jail. He's here and she's not. He goes to her grave and sits. He got a tattoo with her name on it ... . [Her brother], not knowing what to do said, "We are going to be fine." He moved [away for college]. He was devastated that he wasn't a match [for bone marrow transplantation], only a partial match. He still struggles with it. He is getting married on her birthday. He still struggles with it. We raised them as a team (parent crying).
• It's hard for [our daughter] to say goodbye to anybody now ... . She's better able to talk about him. She used to not be able to.
• These brothers were close from the day they were born ... . If there's psychological problems that you can see happening to them or they're going off the deep end with drugs or alcohol or whatever, you might try to address it ... . We were able to walk away from it. He scared the hell out of his mom.
Grandparent
I think my mom was affected. [Our daughter] was her only grandchild. I think it was really hard. She talks about her all the time.

Parents described their need and their family's need for anticipatory grief counseling. Parents described having become so engaged with their ill child that they neglected other family roles and responsibilities: "Right before [our son] died, [our daughter was] ... vandalizing school, ... throwing mud, ... piercing her own ears, like self-mutilation." Parents were unable to support their other children and spouse. In retrospect, participants wished that all family members had received anticipatory bereavement services.

COMMUNICATION

The third primary theme was *communication*. Examples of parents' comments are noted in Table 6. Participants had appreciated the provider's time for discussion and understood that a provider's availability fluxed in accordance with the child's health status. Participants needed providers to lead end-of-life conversations:

> [Our son's doctor] did it well. We never had false hope. [The doctor said], "This is what we can try. I'll tell you what we are accustomed to seeing,

TABLE 6 Theme: Communication

- [When the tumor] spread, we knew … that it was the beginning of the end. Maybe we should have talked about it then and not waited until the end. Why would you wait until the end for something that you know is coming?
- [One] doctor said, "I have other patients," implying my daughter was not a priority. That's why we are here [at the focus group], so no one has to feel the way we feel.
- "Read this book, and if you need anything call us" … . The initiative was all put on us.
- [At home], I remember a few times being frustrated, being so far away, trying to reach somebody and not being able to get [the doctor]. We didn't know who to call or talk to. We had emergencies about vomiting.
- [The staff asked], "What do you want to know?", and we're going, "We don't know what to ask."
- He had these appointments but we didn't know why. [We need to know the] medical reason for the visit.
- He was terminal. [While he was resting, my husband] and I went to the cafeteria. When we got back, the physical therapist had him in the chair to do physical therapy and he was having a seizure!
- We were well informed. We knew beforehand that if she relapsed, there was no cure.
- [Our son's doctor] did it well. We never had false hope. [The doctor said], "This is what we can try. I'll tell you what we are accustomed to seeing, as far as [treatment] response" … . [The doctor] took us [aside] and said you need to talk to [your son] about funeral plans … . We didn't tell him right away; he had that summer. But we knew there was a strong possibility [that he would not make it].
- "What aren't you telling me?" I still think there are things they didn't tell us. They said she would be better. Treatment was cut and dry: do [the treatment, then] go home. When they took her to [ICU] … no one ever talked to us, like trying to get blood out of turnip … . If [I knew she was dying], … I would have taken my child home because that's where she wanted to be.
- They took as long as it took. They were never in a hurry to leave our room. We learned to be patient because we knew that those doctors were with other parents and doing the same thing, so we learned to be very patient because we knew they were coming to talk to us.
- There was a lot of negativism. The doctors would say, "He's not moving this. He's not having any kind of actions. We're not sure, blah blah, what's going on" … . He had just come out of a coma. We were communicating with him by eyelid, hand, and toe movements, which the doctors failed to acknowledge. They were talking … about him to us. We told them to stop.
- Each hospitalization was like a brand-new episode. There wasn't good record keeping, communication [from one hospitalization to the next].
- Trust [makes for good communication].
- Communication, record keeping was lacking [between] departments.
- [The doctor] said, "I have to tell you that [your son]'s not gonna [sic] make it." He told us as well as he possibly could … . Some people may not want to know, but for us, we wanted to know as soon as [the doctor knew].
- [Use] layman's terms [like] *supportive care*. Speak English. I've already got this *cancer* word weighing me down. Keep it straight and simple.
- We were prepared to talk about [death]. They were not … . We never got to the part where they said, "Would you want us to talk with [your son]?"
- [Our son] had lost the ability to talk and communicate. We pretty much knew where we were but no one … told us. I finally called a time out and said, "I'd like to speak to you doctor" … . I felt no one was ready and available. I had to ask the question … . We gotta [sic] know. The name [palliative care] should be changed. I would have never known what it was if I didn't put 2 and 2 together. It's not a word we use in everyday life. It's a foreign word to me.
- Extracting information from the doctors, a very sensitive subject for me … . The end-of-life issues were probably the biggest.

TABLE 7 Themes: Social Support, Decision Making, Spiritual Care, and Symptom Management

---

Social support
- [His brother] would come up on the weekends, stay with him, give us a break, let us get out, have some social time to ourselves, trade off with grandparents, friends.
- He wanted to be with his friends and in class as much as possible …. I would wheel him out [and] put him in the car—literally pick him up and put him in the driver's seat, put the wheelchair in the back. He would drive to school, call his buddies from class and say, "Hey, I'm in the parking lot. Can you come get me?" … Tons of support in every teacher, principal and student.
- My daughter wanted her friends.
- We like talking about [our son], and we like people listening …. I've let everybody know, "Don't ever feel like you've reminded me that I've lost my son. I think about him constantly, all the time, so don't ever be afraid to mention him."
- Everybody brought pictures for the visitation. They asked us for his trophies and letter jacket. The entire gymnasium was decorated, all the way around. Some of the pictures were wall size, 8' × 10', of him in his tux, every phase of his life. A CD [of him] was playing.
- You come here and meet everyone and know about their life and then you go home …. [I] get on Facebook. I am friends with all of [my daughter's] nurses.
- Families and kids need a network to call from the beginning. We need to hear, "You aren't weird. Do what works for you." You can't always talk to friends. You cry, and they think they should fix it and fear offending you. [Friends] just need to let me be a mess.
- There should be a fundraiser for parents [left with] bills.

Decision making
- Hospice was … an abrupt transition …. We were talking to the doctors here … and then, it was like divorce from the hospital (hand gesture implying they were just kicked out).
- To make a decision, you need information and education …. I want to know, "What is this treatment?" They gave some … information and papers, but it wasn't enough.
- [The doctors] communicated very well. When it came to decision making, they provided the history and all the options, so we had enough information to make a sound decision.
- When it came to palliative care, there was some conflict, some decision they wanted to make that we didn't agree with. We did voice our opinion. In most cases it was [respected]. I think there were one or two instances where it was not.

Spiritual care
- A pastor came by all the time. Couldn't ask for anything better.
- [A chaplain we did not know] came in right after [the doctor] tells us [our son] is going to die …. That was not a good time …. [The doctor] probably should have said, "Would you like to have a chaplain come by?" That would've been different. At that point, we just wanted each other.

Symptom management
- [In pediatrics,] we were introduced to palliative care immediately. We had been [with the adult service] for over a year and didn't know there was any such thing as palliative care. We could have used that earlier …. [Our son] only had one fear—that was his lungs filling up with fluid …. He said, "I can handle the cancer …. I just cannot handle not being able to breathe" …. It happened a couple of times and that scared him. That's the only time he ever got scared, when he couldn't catch his breath. The pediatrician explained palliative care, and [our son] understood it perfectly, and we were all going, "Wow, that's a great idea. I can't believe nobody's introduced this to us before."
- [My son] had a lot of pain. The [staff] did a wonderful job.

> as far as [treatment] response" ... . [The doctor] took us [aside] and said you need to talk to [your son] about funeral plans ... . We didn't tell him right away; he had that summer. But we knew there was a strong possibility [that he would not make it].

At transitional treatment points, parents lacked knowledge and related experience and had not known enough to formulate relevant questions. The word "extraction" was used by parents to describe the extraordinary effort necessary to garner prognostic information.

A sense of "seamlessness" in treatment plan and across providers, departments, and hospitalizations had been desired. If a disconnection or interruption occurred in the treatment plan or process, parents monitored and informed providers. If the disconnection was not quickly remedied, parents became hyper-vigilant and felt insecure leaving the child unattended: "He was terminal. [While he was resting, my husband] and I went to the cafeteria. When we got back, the physical therapist had him in the chair to do physical therapy and he was having a seizure!" This vigilant, defensive posture kindled parental anxiety.

SOCIAL SUPPORT

Representative quotations regarding social support, decision making, spiritual care, and symptom management are provided in Table 7. *Social support*, the need to maintain social relationships and connections with local community members, had not been an identified content domain through the literature review conducted at the time of the interview script development. Sustaining a locally based community support system was highly valued:

> He wanted to be with his friends and in class as much as possible ... . I would wheel him out [and] put him in the car—literally pick him up and put him in the driver's seat, put the wheelchair in the back. He would drive to school, call his buddies from class and say, "Hey, I'm in the parking lot. Can you come get me?" ... Tons of support in every teacher, principal and student.

Parents emphasized the importance of discussing social support needs with providers and maximizing social connections in the treatment plan.

DISCUSSION

Consistent themes were found among parents of diverse backgrounds whose children were of different cancer diagnoses. Parents appeared grateful to have an opportunity to tell their children's stories, validate the lives of their children, confirm the importance of service providers, and express their concerns in a nonjudgmental environment. They wanted to give feedback to the treatment providers who gave so much and to rectify wrongs for future children and families.

Standards of care, emotional care, communication, and social support were focal areas of interest for participants. Of the emergent domains, two had been identified in the literature review and through expert consultations: the emotional care of family members and communication between family members and providers. These themes were supported by previous studies (Hinds, Oakes, Hicks, & Anghelescu, 2005; Meert et al., 2008; Klassen, Gulati, & Dix, 2012). Meyer and colleagues highlighted the importance of family-provider communication (Meyer, Ritholz, Burns, & Truog, 2006). In the sample from Kreicbergs, Valdimarsdottir, Onelov, Henter, and Steineck, (2004), parents valued accessible staff coordinated care and consistent information regarding their child's disease, treatment, decision making, and death. These studies suggested that discussions with the child, parents, and providers are particularly critical toward the end of life. Parents needed to know what to expect and how to prepare (Hinds et al., 1996; Mack et al., 2005). Yet the findings from a retrospective medical record review by Zhukovsky, Herzog, Kaur, Palmer, & Bruera (2009) suggested that in clinical practice, discussions of this nature are rare. Further research on the cause or the "disconnect" between established professional standards and appropriate intervention can guide future directions for pediatric palliative clinical practice.

Parents in this study stressed the importance of establishing long-term relationships and effective communication with their child's health care providers. The inverse has been discussed in the literature. Providers feel rewarded when close and trusting relationships with parents and children endured throughout the child's care (Klassen, Gulati, & Dix, 2012; Meert et al., 2008). The close, trusting relationships may help navigate unique combinations of variables encountered throughout treatment and death. The idiosyncrasies of individuals, illnesses and their natural history, and their numerous treatment environments occur in infinite combinations. Close relationships accommodate the dynamic and personal nature of this process. Many of the suggestions made by these parents applied to both primary oncology and palliative care and were not limited to one time segment in the child's life. The level of importance ascribed to particular aspects of care varied according to time, experience, and health status. A trajectory of serious illness may be unpredictable and the needs of children and families are dynamic. Priorities of care should be reassessed as the child's health condition changes.

Two primary areas of interest to participants were standards of care and social support. Failure to meet some of the patients and families' basic needs highlighted issues specific to treating children within the context of subspecialty adult clinics and inpatient units. The structure of the tertiary comprehensive cancer center that was the recruitment site for this study, a children's hospital within a subspecialty, adult hospital, appeared to have contributed to some of the unique standard of care issues described. This particular study findings provides important institution-specific feedback for improving the quality of PPC provided by this institution.

The role of social support in both mental and physical health has long been established (Baron, Cutrona, Hicklin, Russell, & Lubaroff, 1990; Cutrona, Russell, & Rose, 1986; Cutrona, Cole, Colangelo, Assouline, & Russell, 1994; Russell & Cutrona, 1991). The participants in this study stressed the critical importance of social support during the course of a child's serious illness. The need for long-standing friendships and connection with one's local community and its members was considered essential. Social support or being anchored by one's local community in the sanctuary of friendship was defined by this sample as a core element to coping, prior to and following their child's death.

Study Limitations

Limitations of this study include the small sample size, limited generalizability, sample selection bias, and recall bias. First, the number of parents who participated in the focus groups was small but acceptable for a qualitative study and a sensitive topic. Despite the small sample size, the participants were engaged and provided meaningful feedback.

The focus groups were conducted in a large tertiary cancer center with a breadth of available resources, standards, policies, and algorithms of care. Some results of from this study may not be generalizable to other populations of children receiving palliative care in community hospitals, for example. Clinicians should be cautious when generalizing to other clinical settings or populations.

Sample selection bias was another study limitation. Participants were exclusively parents. Needs, barriers, and quality of care are perceived differently depending on the personal perspective (child, parent, or provider). Providers tend to focus on biomedical factors such as treatment planning, while parents focus on the nature of provider communication (Mack et al., 2005). Parents characterize quality communication as being collaborative, family-centered, honest, complete, and sensitive, caring in manner of delivery (Feudtner, 2007; Jones, 2005; Kovacs, Bellin, & Fauri, 2006). Parents advocated in accordance with what other investigators have learned directly from children. Children who have the opportunity to discuss their illness and related concerns tend to feel less anxious and isolated (Hurwitz, Duncan, & Wolfe, 2004; Institute of Medicine, 2003a, 2003b) and benefit emotionally from participating in treatment decision making (Wolfe, Friebert, & Hilden, 2002). Research indicates that when children participate in health-related conversations and decision making, they can make meaningful contributions (Hinds et al., 2005; Wolfe et al., 2002).

A fourth limitation was recall bias of the experiences reported by bereaved parents during the focus groups. How time between their child's death and the focus groups may have affected parents' recall is unclear. Several parents described the memory of their child as being with them "constantly." One parent shared that "I've let everybody know, 'don't ever feel like you've reminded me that I've lost my son.' I think about him constantly, all the time, so don't ever be afraid to mention him." The extent to which recall bias tainted subject matter of this emotional valence is unclear and deserves consideration in future study designs.

CLINICAL PRACTICE IMPLICATIONS

Social workers, by nature of their profession, work with human emotions on a daily basis; with families who come from a variety of cultural, socioeconomic, or spiritual backgrounds; and with individuals confronting numerous personal challenges simultaneously. Thus, a characteristic integral to social workers rests upon the emotional intelligence required of a profession that serves the most vulnerable populations in society, including families dealing with the death of a family member. Emotional intelligence has been defined "as a core aptitude related to one's ability and capacity to reason with one's emotions, especially in relation to others" (Freshwater & Stickley, 2004, p. 92). The combination of a social worker's emotional intelligence, professional training, and experiential knowledge provides a strong foundation for dealing with the emotions that accompany the potential or actual death of a child; developing open and trusting communication with children, families, and providers; serving as a negotiator or advocate as needed; and building therapeutic relationships with children who are at the end of life and their families.

The results of this study have implications for social work models of practice, standards of care, educational curriculum, and research. Feedback from bereaved parents provided unexpected insights on PPC, and emphasized the importance and desired characteristics of patient-provider interactions. Parents also stressed the importance of having someone from the team contact the parents after the child's death. Parents expressed feeling abandoned and not having access to providers who had known their child or understood the intensity of the emotional journey that the parents and families had just completed or, in some instances, were still experiencing. Social workers are well prepared to offer support to parents, siblings, and other family members through grief/bereavement services or support groups and to identify resources that would provide bereavement counseling in their local communities.

Study results pertaining to communication and emotional support could be applied in the course of advance care planning with parents and children. Legacy activities, documenting preferences for medical and nonmedical care, supporting decisions made related to resuscitation status, and symptom management advocacy are key components of social work services (Orloff, 2011; Jones & Phillips, 2011). The suggestions made by parents have the potential to shape the execution of these job responsibilities.

Social work education and academic curriculum are ideal avenues for introducing palliative and end-of-life standards of care, policies, and model of clinical practice to students or novice social workers early in their professional career. These data may also be used to educate social workers who do not specialize in PPC on the needs of bereaved parents. Professional organizations (e.g., SWHPN, NASW, AOSW) and academic institutions provide continuing education courses, websites to monitor changes in practice, and other social media means that build networks among social workers interested in palliative and end-of life care for children or adults. Future research is warranted to explore how social work assessments and interventions might enhance communication between the child, parent, and providers; increase empowerment and advocacy skills in children and parents; and contribute to the "good death" of a child (Welch, 2008).

CONCLUSION

Parents of children who died from cancer provided candid feedback and best practice suggestions. When and how services were executed at the end of a child's life had a lasting impact on the surviving parents. Many of the suggestions were psychosocial in nature. Social workers are professionally trained and equipped to provide what the parents desired. The parents' distillation of and direction in applying the skills serve to complement the social worker's formal training and give credibility to initiatives, direction, and leadership taken by the medical team's social worker. Social workers are encouraged to integrate this evidence into practice for the delivery of optimal pediatric palliative and end-of-life care.

REFERENCES

Altilio, T., Gardia, G., & Otis-Green, S. (2007). Social work practice in palliative and end-of-life care: A report from the summit. *Journal of Social Work in End-of-Life and Palliative Care, 3*(4), 68–86.

Altilio, T., & Otis-Green, S. (2005). "Res Ipsa Loquitur" ... it speaks for itself ... social work-values, pain, and palliative care. *Journal of Social Work in End-of-Life and Palliative Care, 1*(4), 3–6.

Altilio, T., Otis-Green, S., & Dahlin, C. M. (2008). Applying the National Quality Forum Preferred Practices for Palliative and Hospice Care: A social work perspective. *Journal of Social Work in End-of-Life and Palliative Care, 4*(1), 3–16. doi:10.1080/15524250802071999

Association of Pediatric Oncology Social Workers. (2005). *Core elements in pediatric palliative care*. Retrieved from http://www.aposw.org

Baron, R. S., Cutrona, C. E., Hicklin, D., Russell, D. W., & Lubaroff, D. M. (1990). Social support and immune function among spouses of cancer patients. *Journal of Personality and Social Psychology, 59*(2), 344–352.

Bern-Klug, M., Kramer, B. J., & Linder, J. F. (2005). All aboard: Advancing the social work research agenda in end-of-life and palliative care. *Journal of Social Work in End-of-Life and Palliative Care, 1*(2), 71–86.

Christ, G., & Blacker, S. (2006). Shaping the future of social work in end-of-life and palliative care. *Journal of Social Work in End-of-Life and Palliative Care, 2*(1), 5–12. doi:10.1300/J457v02n01_02

Creswell, J. W. (2006). *Qualitative inquiry and research design: Choosing among five approaches* (2nd ed.). Thousand Oaks, CA: Sage.

Cutrona, C., Russell, D., & Rose, J. (1986). Social support and adaptation to stress by the elderly. *Psychology and Aging, 1*(1), 47–54.

Cutrona, C. E., Cole, V., Colangelo, N., Assouline, S. G., & Russell, D. W. (1994). Perceived parental social support and academic achievement: An attachment theory perspective. *Journal of Personality and Social Psychology, 66*(2), 369–378.

Feudtner, C. (2007). Collaborative communication in pediatric palliative care: A foundation for problem-solving and decision-making. *Pediatric Clinics of North America, 54*(5), 583–607, ix. doi:S0031-3955(07)00117-4 [pii]10.1016/j.pcl. 2007.07.008

Foster, T. L., Lafond, D. A., Reggio, C., & Hinds, P. S. (2010). Pediatric palliative care in childhood cancer nursing: From diagnosis to cure or end of life. *Seminars in Oncology Nursing, 26*(4), 205–221. doi:S0749-2081(10)00050-1 [pii]10.1016/j. soncn.2010.08.003

Freshwater, D., & Stickley, T. (2004). The heart of the art: Emotional intelligence in nurse education. *Nursing Inquiry, 11*(2), 91–98. doi:10.1111/j.1440-1800.2004. 00198.xNIN198 [pii]

Gwyther, L. P., Altilio, T., Blacker, S., Christ, G., Csikai, E. L., Hooyman, N., … Howe, J. (2005). Social work competencies in palliative and end-of-life care. *Journal of Social Work in End-of-Life and Palliative Care, 1*(1), 87–120. doi:10.1300/ J457v01n01_06

Hinds, P. S., Birenbaum, L. K., Clarke-Steffen, L., Quargnenti, A., Kreissman, S., Kazak, A., … Wilimas, J. (1996). Coming to terms: Parents' response to a first cancer recurrence in their child. *Nursing Research, 45*(3), 148–153.

Hinds, P. S., Drew, D., Oakes, L. L., Fouladi, M., Spunt, S. L., Church, C., & Furman, W. L. (2005). End-of-life care preferences of pediatric patients with cancer. *Journal of Clinical Oncology, 23*(36), 9146–9154. doi:JCO.2005.10.538 [pii]

Hinds, P. S., Oakes, L. L., Hicks, J., & Anghelescu, D. L. (2005). End-of-life care for children and adolescents. *Seminars in Oncology Nursing, 21*(1), 53–62.

Hurwitz, C. A., Duncan, J., & Wolfe, J. (2004). Caring for the child with cancer at the close of life: "There are people who make it, and I'm hoping I'm one of them". *JAMA, 292*(17), 2141–2149. doi:292/17/2141 [pii]10.1001/jama.292.17.2141

Institute of Medicine. (2003a). Communication, goal setting, and care planning. In M. Field, & R. Behrman (Eds.), *When children die: Improving palliative and end of life care for children and their families* (pp. 104–140). Washington, DC: The National Academies Press.

Institute of Medicine. (2003b). *When children die: Improving palliative and end-of-life care for children and their families*. Washington, DC: The National Academies Press.

Jones, B. L. (2005). Pediatric palliative and end-of-life care: The role of social work in pediatric oncology. *Journal of Social Work in End-of-Life and Palliative Care, 1*(4), 35–61.

Jones, B. L., & Phillips, F. (2011). *Social work in pediatric palliative care* (1st ed.). New York, NY: Oxford University Press.

Klassen, A., Gulati, S., & Dix, D. (2012). Health care providers' perspectives about working with parents of children with cancer: A qualitative study. *Journal of Pediatric Oncology Nursing, 29*(2), 92–97 doi:10.1177/1043454212438405

Kovacs, P. J., Bellin, M. H., & Fauri, D. P. (2006). Family-centered care: A resource for social work in end-of-life and palliative care. *Journal of Social Work in End-of-Life and Palliative Care, 2*(1), 13–27. doi:10.1300/J457v02n01_03

Kramer, B. J., Christ, G. H., Bern-Klug, M., & Francoeur, R. B. (2005). A national agenda for social work research in palliative and end-of-life care. *Journal of Palliative Medicine, 8*(2), 418–431. doi:10.1089/jpm.2005.8.418

Kreicbergs, U., Valdimarsdottir, U., Onelov, E., Henter, J. I., & Steineck, G. (2004). Talking about death with children who have severe malignant disease. *New England Journal of Medicine, 351*(12), 1175–1186. doi:10.1056/NEJMoa 040366351/12/1175 [pii]

Mack, J. W., Hilden, J. M., Watterson, J., Moore, C., Turner, B., Grier, H. E., … Wolfe, J. (2005). Parent and physician perspectives on quality of care at the end of life in children with cancer. *Journal of Clinical Oncology, 23*(36), 9155–9161. doi:JCO.2005.04.010 [pii]10.1200/JCO.2005.04.010

Mayan, M. J. (2001). *An introduction to qualitative methods. International Institute for Qualitative Methodology*. Edmonton, AB, Canada: Qual Institute Press.

Meert, K. L., Eggly, S., Pollack, M., Anand, K. J., Zimmerman, J., Carcillo, J., … Nicholson, C. (2008). Parents' perspectives on physician-parent communication near the time of a child's death in the pediatric intensive care unit. *Pediatric Critical Care Medicine, 9*(1), 2–7. doi:10.1097/01.PCC.0000298644.13882.88

Meyer, E. C., Ritholz, M. D., Burns, J. P., & Truog, R. D. (2006). Improving the quality of end-of-life care in the pediatric intensive care unit: Parents' priorities and recommendations. *Pediatrics, 117*(3), 649–657. doi:117/3/649 [pii]10.1542/peds.2005-0144

Miles, M. B. (1994). *Qualitative data analysis: An expanded sourcebook* (2nd ed.). Thousand, Oaks, CA: Sage.

Morgan, D. L. (1993). *Successful focus groups: Advancing the state of the art*. Thousand Oaks, CA: Sage.

National Association of Social Workers. (2004). *NASW standards for palliative and end of life care*. Retrieved from http://www.naswdc.org/practice/bereavement/standards/default.asp

Orloff, S. F. (2011). *Pediatric hospice and palliative care: The invaluable role of social work*. New York, NY: Oxford University Press.

Palos, G. (2011). *Social work research agenda in palliative and end-of-life care* (1st ed.). New York, NY: Oxford University Press.

Russell, D. W., & Cutrona, C. E. (1991). Social support, stress, and depressive symptoms among the elderly: Test of a process model. *Psychology and Aging, 6*(2), 190–201.

Welch, S. B. (2008). Can the death of a child be good? *Journal of Pediatric Nursing*, *23*(2), 120–125. doi:S0882-5963(07)00332-6 [pii]10.1016/j.pedn.2007.08.015

Wolfe, J., Friebert, S., & Hilden, J. (2002). Caring for children with advanced cancer integrating palliative care. *Pediatric Clinics of North America*, *49*(5), 1043–1062.

Zhukovsky, D. S., Herzog, C. E., Kaur, G., Palmer, J. L., & Bruera, E. (2009). The impact of palliative care consultation on symptom assessment, communication needs, and palliative interventions in pediatric patients with cancer. *Journal of Palliative Medicine*, *12*(4), 343–349. doi:10.1089/jpm.2008.0152

"I'll Never Forget Those Cold Words as Long as I Live": Parent Perceptions of Death Notification for Stillbirth

SUZANNE PULLEN

Hugh Downs School of Human Communication, Arizona State University, Tempe, Arizona, USA

MINDI ANN GOLDEN

Communication Studies, San Francisco State University, San Francisco, California, USA

JOANNE CACCIATORE

School of Social Work, Arizona State University, Phoenix, Arizona, USA

This qualitative study analyzed stillbirth notification messages recalled by parents who strongly agreed (n = 47) and strongly disagreed (n = 43) that the way news about the death of their infant was delivered negatively impacted their grieving process. Three message elements formed a core stillbirth notification experience (delay of news delivery; expression of sympathy; communication of death), and three additional message elements occurred in both data sets (communication regarding options; expression of uncertainty; exit of health care provider); however, the messages differed in form and frequency between the two groups. Three message elements reflected opposing experiences for the two groups (support of parent emotion; continuity of care; and information provision). Recommendations for stillbirth notification that emphasize acknowledging parent perceptions, clear language and information, empathetic communication, and continuity of care are given.

Walking into her doctor's office for a prenatal visit, a healthy mother-to-be, having experienced no complications in her pregnancy does not expect to hear the words, "Your baby's heart has stopped beating." In the United States, words like these convey the devastating news of stillbirth more than 25,000 times every year (MacDorman & Kirmeyer, 2009). Stillbirth is an emotionally and physiologically painful and traumatic event that occurs suddenly and often without warning (Cacciatore & Bushfield, 2007; Gold, 2007). A deep sense of attachment often develops between a mother and unborn child during pregnancy; thus, she is likely to experience profound psychological distress, including high risk of posttraumatic stress disorder (PTSD) upon the baby's death (Cacciatore & Bushfield, 2007; Trulsson & Radestad, 2004). Mothers' grief experiences following the death of a baby to stillbirth are further complicated by the biological fact of death occurring within the body; cultural discomfort with death, particularly a child's death; and feelings of anxiety, failure, and guilt (Cacciatore, 2010; Condon, 1986; Reddy, 2007).

Because many health care providers (HCPs) are often uncomfortable when a patient dies, particularly when the patient is a baby or a child, support for parents experiencing stillbirth may be compromised (Gold, 2007). Obstetric nurses and physicians receive a dearth of death education, and generally feel unprepared to face the profound losses of a baby's death (Cacciatore & Bushfield, 2007; Chan, Chan, & Day, 2003; Säflund, Sjögren, & Wredling, 2002).

However, parents do report that HCPs' behavior and their handling of stillbirth is important to their experiences of loss (Gold, 2007; Säflund, Sjörgen, & Wredling, 2004). When bereaved parents perceive HCPs as dishonest and not forthcoming, they experience increased anxiety and mistrust toward their providers (Schott, Henley, & Kohner, 2007). Parents also report being upset by care provider behaviors perceived as avoidant, insensitive, and lacking in emotional support. Conversely, when medical professionals are perceived as caring and honest, patients report feelings of appreciation despite their tragic circumstances (Gold, 2007).

Physicians have identified conversations with parents experiencing the death of a baby as more serious than conversations with patients about any other condition (Säflund, 2003), and a few studies have examined HCP opinions of, treatment plans for, or conversations with parents experiencing stillbirth (Chan et al., 2003; Kirkley-Best, Kellner, & Ladue, 1984–1985; Robson, Thompson, & Ellwood, 2006; Säflund et al., 2002). However, no studies to date have examined perceptions of death notification in the context of stillbirth. In addition, despite research showing the value of empathy in provider-patient communication and efforts to improve communication during medical training (Ahrens & Hart, 1997; Benenson & Pollack, 2003; Levetown, 2008), there has been little change in patient perceptions of doctors as less supportive than nurses (Gold, 2007). It is critical that health care providers develop a clearer understanding of how death notification can impact a patient's grieving process, both positively and negatively.

DEATH NOTIFICATION

HCPs describe death notification (i.e., telling persons that their loved one has died) as emotional and indicate that delivering news of a child's death is especially unsettling (Clark & LaBeff, 1982). Ahrens and Hart (1997) found that HCPs believed the experience of communicating the news of a child's death was the most difficult experience in emergency medicine, more difficult than communicating the death of an adult to his or her family. Some HCPs find the death of a baby or child so distressing that they shy away from empathizing with the parent(s) (Leon, 1992). HCPs struggle with how much emotion to show when delivering news of the death, how to deliver the news (e.g., direct telling may be perceived as cold), and how to respond to the family member's reactions (Clark & LaBeff, 1982).

HCPs also report feeling unprepared to engage in death notification due to lack of education or training (Ahrens & Hart, 1997; Benenson & Pollack, 2003; Hobgood, Tamayo-Sarver, Hollar, & Sawning, 2009; Leash, 1996; Smith-Cumberland & Feldman, 2006; Stewart, Lord, & Mercer, 2000). However, when HCPs receive death notification education, the training appears to improve confidence in their ability to deliver news of death (Nordström, 2011; Ponce et al., 2010; Smith-Cumberland, 2006; Smith-Cumberland & Feldman, 2006). However, some assert that death education focused on psychosocial care can be problematic if it encourages adherence to a fixed protocol or sequence of steps that do not account for individual patient responses, nuances, and needs (Cacciatore & Flint, 2012; Villagran, Goldsmith, Wittenberg-Lyles, & Baldwin, 2010).

Little extant research has explored bereaved parents' perspectives about what is helpful during death notification (Gyulay, 1989; Janzen, Cadell, & Westhues, 2003–2004). However, interactions with HCPs do influence bereaved parents. For example, negative interactions exacerbate trauma symptomology while compassionate caring promotes positive outcomes for grieving parents (Janzen et al., 2003–2004). Also, parents whose children die suddenly report wanting their doctors to show compassion, give information, explain procedures, and provide support referrals (Janzen et al., 2003–2004). Parents prefer that HCPs demonstrate a caring attitude and allow them to express their emotions (Gold, 2007; Levetown, 2008). Getting inadequate or poorly delivered information (Levetown, 2008; Schott et al., 2007), receiving conflicting opinions from multiple HCPs (Levetown, 2008), experiencing delay of death notification (Leash, 1996), and hearing jargon-laden or indirect terminology (Prasad, 2010) can negatively impact the way bereaved parents perceive HCP communication.

The literature suggests that interactions with HCPs have a profound impact on parents who experience a perinatal death. Even years after being told that their baby is stillborn, parents are clear that some communication from health care providers helped them and some communication still leaves them feeling angry and upset (Fallowfield & Jenkins, 2004; Gold 2007). How the death of a baby to stillbirth is communicated may impact satisfaction with care provision, a parent's sense of social support, and the severity of long-term psychological distress (Trulsson & Radestad, 2004). Hence, given the dearth of literature published on this subject, the purpose of this study was to describe how notification following the death of a baby to stillbirth is recalled by patients and how that communication impacted their grieving process. Specifically, the research question guiding this study was: What death notification message elements were recalled by parents with strong feelings about how news of their baby's death to stillbirth was delivered?

METHOD

A retrospective study, using an IRB-approved questionnaire regarding parent perceptions of perinatal loss diagnosis delivery was administered via an online survey service (SurveyMonkey). Data analyzed in this study are part of a larger project regarding communication in the context of stillbirth. The questionnaire contained open- and closed-ended questions. The first author, having experienced the death of a baby to stillbirth, is active in various support communities for bereaved parents; thus, participants were recruited and contacted through participation and membership in organizations that offer services to bereaved parents of perinatal loss.

Sample

Anyone who had a perinatal death was allowed to complete the survey, but this study focused only on data collected from participants who reported their diagnosis was stillbirth. This was defined as the intrauterine death of a baby 20 weeks gestation or greater ($n = 624$). Females accounted for 97.4% ($n = 599$) of respondents, with 97.9% ($n = 597$) self-identified as heterosexual, and 83.2% ($n = 510$) self-identified as married.

Measures and Data Analysis

For the purpose of this study, all surveys of participants who had experienced stillbirth wherein respondents strongly agreed that they recalled the exact words a health care provider used to deliver death notifications were selected ($n = 222$). These data were then sorted on the basis of either strong agreement or strong disagreement with the survey item, "The way I found out about the diagnosis negatively impacted my grieving process." Fifty-one respondents strongly agreed and 47 strongly disagreed.

From the 98 surveys, those in which the participant also responded to the open-ended item "Please write down what the care provider said and/or did when s/he delivered the news of the diagnosis" were selected (50 of 51 and 45 of 47 respondents, respectively). Upon review, five surveys were eliminated because how the parent was told the baby died was not included or the description indicated that a live birth had occurred. Hence, messages reported by 47 parents who strongly agreed and 43 parents who strongly disagreed that the death notification negatively impacted their grieving process were analyzed.

Data were analyzed using a constant comparison method associated with grounded theory (Glaser & Strauss, 1968). The first step was open coding. This involved the first and second authors independently reading each death notification description, identifying distinct message elements, and then discussing what they had identified in order to achieve negotiated consensus. As in Salander's (2002) research, message descriptions differed in that some participants only provided the words they recalled a HCP using to deliver death notification (e.g., "I'm sorry, both your babies are dead"), while others described a sequence of events constituting the larger process of news delivery (e.g., "The nurse then told me she was going to get another Doppler to find the heart beat maybe this one is broke"). In all cases, what Strauss and Corbin (1990) term discreet incidents or ideas were identified and labeled. For example, "I'm sorry, both your babies are dead" contains two discreet ideas—an expression of sympathy and communication of death.

The second, interrelated step in data analysis was axial coding, which focuses on connections between categories (Strauss & Corbin, 1990). Specifically, subcategories were linked to categories, with particular regard to communication strategies and consequences (Strauss & Corbin, 1990). For example, that communication of death occurred was not surprising, but several distinct ways of communicating (i.e., subcategories) were identified. The authors worked through the data line-by-line, examining discreet message elements and asking, "How are these similar and how are these different?" The result was a detailed description of message elements reported by parents who had strong feelings about whether or not the way death notification was delivered negatively impacted their grieving process. For clarity in reporting findings, the two groups are referred to as parents perceiving HCP communication positively and negatively.

FINDINGS

A total of 14 message elements were identified in parent descriptions of recalled diagnosis of stillbirth. Six elements occurred in both data sets (i.e., parents perceiving HCP communication positively or negatively), with three of the six elements forming a core death notification experience. The two groups differed in the form and frequency of these message elements. Three additional message elements in each data set formed bipolar opposites in relation to one another, while five message elements were unique to the group perceiving HCP communication negatively.

A Core Experience in Death Notification for Stillbirth

Parents in both groups commonly described three message elements at the heart of a diagnosis of the baby's death: delay of news delivery, expression of sympathy, and communication of death; however, there were experiential distinctions between the groups (see Appendix 1 for an overview of key differences between the two groups).

DELAY OF NEWS DELIVERY

Following an initial indication of possible death such as a heartbeat not being detected during an ultrasound, a HCP may take additional measures to confirm the diagnosis, thus the process of diagnosing the baby's death is delayed. Both groups reported delay of news delivery due to: (a) multiple diagnostic exams being conducted or additional HCPs being consulted in one location; (b) parent relocation to another exam room or health care facility; and (c) topic avoidance by HCPs. However, topic avoidance distinguished the two groups, with three times as many parents perceiving HCP communication negatively reporting it compared to parents perceiving HCP communication positively.

EXPRESSION OF SYMPATHY

Expressions of sympathy, particularly simple statements such as "I'm sorry," were reported by parents in both groups, with some indicating more than one expression of sympathy by HCPs; however, compared to the negative group, parents perceiving HCP communication positively reported far more simple statements with intensifiers, such as "I'm so sorry," and nonverbal expressions of sympathy, such as personal touch and the HCP expressing emotion. Nonverbal expressions of sympathy were rare in the negative group.

COMMUNICATION OF DEATH

Communication of death was reported in both groups, generally following a delay in news delivery and, if present, an expression of sympathy. Communication of death varied in that it could be: (a) direct—the parent was told that the baby had died; (b) indirect—HCPs communicated with each other regarding the baby's lack of organ activity within hearing of the parent; (c) implied—a parent must infer a diagnosis from a HCP's comment; and/or (d) nonverbal—a parent sees lack of fetal heartbeat on the monitor or the look on a HCP/family member's face and knows the baby is dead.

Direct death notification was commonly reported in both groups and could be further described as: (a) blunt, using statements like "Your baby is dead"; (b) phrased in the negative, saying things like "There's no heartbeat"; or (c) using idiomatic phrases like "Your baby is gone." Indirect communication was rare in both groups. Parents who perceived HCP communication negatively more frequently reported implied statements of death such as, "Sometimes these things just happen," and parents who perceived HCP communication positively reported more nonverbal communication of death; for example, a HCP asking the parent to look at the monitor as nonverbal reinforcement of verbal communication of death.

Shared Experiences in Death Notification

In addition to the core experience, three additional themes occurred in both groups: communication regarding options, expression of uncertainty, and noted exit of the HCP.

COMMUNICATION REGARDING OPTIONS

Parents perceiving HCP communication positively report being offered delivery options, such as one parent's report that the HCP "nicely explained the options to me and we opted for an epidural and I gave birth vaginally," or being given a medical explanation for why options were limited, such as one parent's explanation that the HCP "told me having a C-section would be ill-advised since they knew the baby was already gone and having one when it wasn't necessary would only set a precedent for future pregnancies ... ." In contrast, parents perceiving HCP communication negatively emphasized being told what the next step would be without explanation, such as one parent's statement that she was " ... told [I] will be given pain relief but have to deliver normally."

EXPRESSED UNCERTAINTY BY HCP

Parents from both groups reported that HCPs expressed uncertainty during their diagnosis but the quality of the messages differed. Parents who perceived HCP communication negatively reported that HCPs: (a) expressed uncertainty regarding the physical condition of the baby, with one HCP making a graphic statement regarding the baby's head possibly detaching in utero; (b) expressed uncertainty regarding examination or treatment, such as one HCP being unsure how to operate the ultrasound machine; or (c) paired uncertainty with hopelessness, such as one HCP saying, "There is a 90% chance your baby is no longer alive." Parents perceiving HCP communication positively reported uncertainty being paired with hopefulness, such as a HCP saying, "The baby might just be hiding from the monitor"; or reported that the HCP expressed uncertainty about how to communicate death to the patient, such as one HCP's statement that, "I don't know how to tell you this." Parents in both groups also reported that HCPs expressed uncertainty about why the baby died. However, parents who perceived HCP communication positively reported that the HCP also stated a possible cause or a desire to find a cause of death.

NOTED EXIT OF HCP

Parents from both groups noted that a HCP "left the room" following death notification and did not report the HCP's return, but the character of the exit again differed between the groups. Parents who perceived HCP communication negatively noted that the HCP exited immediately following communication of death. According to one parent, "He told me that sometimes these things just happen then left the room." Other parents who perceived HCP communication positively specified that the HCP who gave the death notification stayed with them for a while before leaving.

Opposing Experiences in Death Notification

Three message elements in each data set represented opposing experiences for parents. Polar differences in the two data sets were: (a) suppression versus support of patient emotion; (b) lack of versus presence of information provision; and (c) lack of versus presence of continuity of care.

SUPPRESSION OF PATIENT EMOTION VERSUS SUPPORT OF PATIENT EMOTION

Parents who perceived death notification more negatively recalled that attempts were made to suppress their emotions. One parent said the HCP told her that someone would call her husband only "after you get control of yourself." Parents with negative perceptions also said that HCPs prevented others from seeing their emotions. For example, one parent noted that she was told to exit through a side door. Although HCPs may have intended to protect the mother, parents in the latter group perceived HCPs as suppressing the public expression of their emotions.

In contrast to emotion suppression, parents who perceived HCP communication positively described support for their emotions. HCP communication took four forms: (a) time/space for feelings, either with the HCP staying with the parent during her emotional reaction or the HCP saying something like "he would let us have a few minutes alone to let this news sink in and that he'd come back and talk about 'getting our little one here'"; (b) enlisting supportive others, such as calling a family member to be with the parent; (c) validation of feelings, such as acknowledging that the death of a baby is emotionally devastating; and (d) relocation, often meaning taking the patient someplace more private. Relocation was framed as being given the opportunity to grieve and supporting emotion, not a means of hiding the patient, as with emotional suppression.

INFORMATION SHARING VERSUS INFORMATION WITHHOLDING

Parents who perceived HCP communication negatively indicated they did not receive information regarding the baby's death or the information they needed to make important decisions. One parent, for example, noted that a HCP told her that her baby would be stillborn but she did not know what that meant for her or the baby. She did not receive any information from the doctor or hospital about what to expect, about her choices for birth, or about social support in the aftermath of her loss. Another parent indicated that her birth choices were not explained, even though the HCP asked her what she wanted to do.

In contrast, parents who perceived HCP communication positively reported information provision that took three forms: (a) explanation, such as, "He answered any questions we had"; (b) information about what to expect or what the next steps were, such as, "The delivery nurse was great at explaining everything that I should expect"; and (c) cause of death, such as, "She explained through the ultrasound, it looked like the baby knotted his cord by turning breech."

LACK OF CONTINUITY OF CARE VERSUS PRESENCE OF CONTINUITY OF CARE

Parents perceiving HCP communication negatively reported lack of continuity of care, such as not seeing the HCP who delivered death notification again. In other words, the HCP may have come into the examination room, told the parent that the baby died, exited immediately, and avoided future contact with the parent. However, parents who perceived HCP communication positively reported continuity in their care during the death notification process. According to one parent, "The midwife remained with me at all times." Parents also reported continuity of care into the future. For example, one parent explained, "He gave us his personal pager and told us to … call him, no matter what time of night."

Unique Message Elements

Parents who perceived negative HCP communication reported five unique message elements. Specifically, parents reported: (a) isolation, such as being left alone for a long period of time or being put in an isolated location; (b) blame, with the HCP suggesting the parent caused the baby's death; (c) contradiction of experience, such as being told that what the parent felt was impossible; and (d) the death of the baby to stillbirth being cast as beneficial, such as one HCP saying he would include the case in a professional publication. The fifth unique message element, reassurance, was reported by one respondent who said an ultrasound technician's reassurance when she began to blame herself for the baby's death contrasted with a physician's "cold" communication. In this case, the contrasting level of empathy between the technician and doctor contributed to negative perceptions.

DISCUSSION

"We spend the better part of a decade learning to wield the unwieldy words of medicine, but the final lesson is knowing when to put them away." (Prasad, 2010, p. 885)

Death notification appears to take many forms after the death of a baby to stillbirth. Even when HCPs utilize similar message elements, such as communication of death, the specific character of the message can differ, such as being told directly or having the death be implied. At the heart of the differences described by the two groups in this study is verbal and nonverbal communication that may or may not convey care, empathy, and understanding (Mager & Andrykowski, 2002; Salander, 2002; Strauss, Sharp, Lorch, & Kachalia, 1995; Yardley, Davis, & Sheldon, 2001). The death of a baby to stillbirth may be the worst news a parent ever receives (Pullen & Nalos, 2009), but how HCPs communicate about the stillbirth can either foster a sense of support for the parent or exacerbate a sense of fragility (Cacciatore & Bushfield, 2007; Trulsson & Radestad, 2004). A HCP's ability and willingness to engage a grieving parent with humility and mindfulness (Cacciatore, 2010; Cacciatore & Flint, 2012; Watson & Gallois, 1998) rather than with detached objectivity appears key to positive perceptions.

A core experience is perceived by both groups in this study, wherein a delay in the diagnosis is followed by an expression of sympathy and communication of death. However, parents who perceived HCP communication negatively were more likely to report death notification delays due to provider topic avoidance. HCPs may operate under a strict protocol regarding who can explicitly confirm the baby's death to a parent (Statham & Dimavicius, 1992), but silence by HCPs when evidence for death is explicit given multiple exams, additional HCPs being consulted, and the inability to find a heartbeat may prolong distress and confusion (Trulsson & Radestad, 2004).

Many parents reporting negative perceptions did not receive a message of sympathy from their HCP and others received only a simple statement of sympathy. Only two of the parents in the negative group reported any nonverbal support, and that nonverbal support was expressed by only one of the multiple HCPs they saw. "I'm sorry," particularly when not accompanied by mindful provider presence, may not be enough to address what more than one parent described as "the worst day of my life." Verbal intensifiers augment simple statements, and nonverbal expressions demonstrate a level of caring commensurate with the magnitude of the parent's grief. Nonverbal signs of support from HCPs—such as crying, hugging, or holding hands—are highly memorable for parents experiencing stillbirth (Peppers & Knapp, 1980). Parent perceptions in this context appear to mirror health care providers' general reports regarding effective and ineffective bad news delivery experiences, wherein nonverbal behaviors such as eye contact and touch are only described in effective incidents, and expressions of empathy distinguish effective and ineffective incidents (Dickson, Hargie, Brunger, & Stapleton, 2002). However, HCPs also acknowledge that touch is atypical in the delivery of "bad news" (Ptacek & Ellison, 2000).

Although death notification was central in this study, the process took various forms, with implicit statements distinguishing the positive and negative groups. Implied statements of death create potential confusion in that the words spoken, such as, "We missed him by a day," do not clearly relate to death or vital organ functions. HCPs may also minimize the significance of the baby's death for the parent with platitudes such as, "You have another child at home." These types of messages occur more frequently in reports provided by parents linking HCP communication to negative impacts on grieving.

The baby's death was most often communicated verbally to parents, but the frequency with which communication of death was paired with at least one expression of sympathy varied widely between the two groups. Only 18 of 47 parents negatively perceiving HCP communication reported any expression of sympathy in conjunction with communication of death whereas 33 of 43 parents positively perceiving HCP communication reported an expression of sympathy with communication of death. Absence of expressions of sympathy, especially nonverbal expressions, may be highly problematic. Some parents in the negative group characterized HCP behavior as "cold" and "insensitive," while those in the positive group characterized their HCP as "sensitive" and "compassionate." The absence of any expression of sympathy may contribute to a negative perception by the parent. For example, one parent reported the following reaction to a statement made by a doctor called in for a second opinion: "The doctor said, 'I concur the demise of the fetus.' I will never forget those cold words as long as I live." The mere reference to a much-wanted and loved baby as "the fetus" indeed feels "cold" and "detached" and fails to acknowledge the depth of the relationship between a mother and her newborn.

Parents report a desire to express their emotions (as opposed to having emotions suppressed by HCPs), continuity in terms of the HCPs treating them, having their questions answered, and information regarding next steps and cause of their baby's death. These preferences are consistent with past findings regarding effective perinatal end-of-life care from both physician and patient perspectives (Cacciatore & Bushfield, 2007; Dickson et al., 2002;

Ptacek & Ellison, 2000; Salander, 2002; Trulsson & Radestad, 2004; Widger & Picot, 2008).

Finally, messages such as isolation, blame, contradiction of experience, and expressed benefit of the baby's death are solely reported as negative HCP communication. No parent wants to be blamed by her HCP for the tragedy or hear that her baby's death will make an interesting case study.

Based on the perceptions of patients in this study, parents who have experienced stillbirth prefer continuity of care wherein HCPs maintain communication from the moment of suspected death throughout any additional examinations to confirm the death. Parents also desire a clear statement of the baby's death accompanied by verbal and nonverbal expressions of sympathy. Parents prefer that the HCP remain present, allowing time and space for emotions and questions, as well as offering and explaining options. Stillbirth is both a diagnosis for one patient (the parent) that requires subsequent, and often immediate, decision making (e.g., induction of delivery) and death notification regarding a second patient (the child). The traumatic impact of this dual notification requires care and support for the surviving patient in the hours and days following death notification.

Specifically, the findings in this study support many recommendations in competent and compassionate death notification. When a heartbeat is not detected during a routine ultrasound, topic avoidance should not prevail when there are obvious nonverbal signs, such as additional tests and HCPs being consulted, that something is not right. Being aware of the parent's emotional, verbal, and nonverbal response during this time is crucial. If parents are exhibiting signs of anxiety, fear, or a need for information that the technician or nurse cannot provide, rather than ignoring the parent or deflecting the reality of the situation, the HCP can: (a) acknowledge the parent's feeling, perhaps saying, "I can see you are concerned" or "I can image that this might feel stressful"; (b) assure the parent that everything is being done to ascertain the baby's condition by saying something like, "I'm going to get another technician/ doctor here to help me interpret what I'm seeing" or "I need to get another machine to get a better look"; (c) confirm that the parent will get the information as soon as it is possible, perhaps saying, "I'm going to step out and talk with the doctor who will back here in just a few minutes to talk with you and answer any questions you have"; and (d) support the parent by asking if there is anything she needs while waiting to get the results of the exam, saying something such as, "Can I call a partner or a friend to wait with you?"

When the baby's death has been confirmed, the expression of heartfelt sympathy, including nonverbal connection, is important. Also vital is the clear communication of stillbirth that is not cloaked in clinical jargon. Spending time with the grieving mother and creating space for emotional expression is recommended. And, when the parent is ready, psychoeducation about the birth process and alerting parents to their options are helpful and may minimize irremediable regret. Continuity of care is also significant to stillbirth parents. If the clinical setting does not enable the physician determining and/ or delivering stillbirth news to remain with the mother, an interdisciplinary approach wherein a bereavement specialist or social worker trained in death notification is present is recommended to provide comfort, answer questions, and address concerns. Even when the physician is able to remain present, it may be advisable to have a bereavement specialist or social worker present to help parents process both the medical information and the emotional trauma of their baby's death. Just as social workers are not trained to provide diagnoses or perform medical procedures, physicians generally are not trained to help parents navigate the profound psychosocial and spiritual issues of stillbirth the way a bereavement specialist or social worker might.

Limitations and Future Research

In this study, our focus was on parents who strongly agreed or disagreed that the way stillbirth was communicated by HCPs negatively impacted their grieving process. It is possible that focusing on parents with the strongest reactions captures potentially unusual circumstances. Future research can include the parents who did not have such strong reactions about the way stillbirth notification affected their grieving process. A broader look at participant responses might confirm differences and recommendations identified in this research, and also reveal additional strong points of distinction between the groups.

Respondents in this study also provided different types of answers to the open-ended survey item regarding what a HCP said or did during death notification, with some providing the statement of diagnosis and others offering detailed descriptions of events. Future researchers might interview parents in order to derive extended narratives from all participants. This could affirm or extend the findings described in this study, and potentially allow for quantitative distinctions regarding the frequency of message elements experienced by the two groups.

Future research can also build on descriptions of patient perceptions by empirically testing the impacts of message elements. Simulations involving different combinations of preferred and not preferred message elements can be created with observers rating HCPs in terms of empathy, likeability, person-centeredness, and competence. Such research would allow for correlations between specific message elements, or combinations of elements, and perceptions of HCPs and stillbirth notification.

CONCLUSIONS

Based on the results of this study, a HCP's ability to maintain humility, compassion, and mindfulness in the face of a baby's death may diminish short- and long-term negative consequences for parents (Cacciatore & Flint, 2012).

The death of a baby to stillbirth is a devastating experience that has immediate and ongoing emotional, psychological, and social consequences for a family. While HCPs may not be able to predict or prevent many of these deaths, they have a responsibility to mitigate the trauma around the death notification experience for the grieving mother and her family. Ultimately, the onus of the responsibility to *do no harm* falls upon the HCPs. There may be nothing that can ameliorate a parent's natural grieving process, but HCPs can mitigate psychological damage and avoid further exacerbating the trauma.

REFERENCES

Ahrens, W., & Hart, R. (1997). Emergency physicians' experience with pediatric death. *American Journal Of Emergency Medicine, 15*, 642–643.

Benenson, R., & Pollack, M. (2003). Evaluation of emergency medicine resident death notification skills by direct observation. *Academic Emergency Medicine, 10*, 219–223.

Cacciatore, J. (2010). Stillbirth: Clinical recommendations for care in the era of evidence-based medicine. *Clinical Obstetrics and Gynecology, 53*(3), 691–699.

Cacciatore, J., & Bushfield, S. (2007). Stillbirth: The mother's experience and implications for improving care. *Journal of Social Work in End-of-Life & Palliative Care, 3*(3), 59–79.

Cacciatore, J., & Flint, M. (2012). ATTEND: A mindfulness-based bereavement care model. *Death Studies, 36*(1), 61–82.

Chan, M. F., Chan, S. H., & Day, M. C. (2003). Nurses' attitudes towards perinatal bereavement support in Hong Kong: A pilot study. *Journal of Clinical Nursing, 12*, 536–543.

Clark, R. E., & LaBeff, E. E. (1982). Death telling: Managing the delivery of bad news. *Journal of Health and Social Behavior, 23*, 366–380.

Condon, J. T. (1986). Management of established pathological grief reaction after stillbirth. *American Journal of Psychiatry, 143*, 987–992.

Dickson, D., Hargie, O., Brunger, K., & Stapleton, K. (2002). Health professionals' perceptions of breaking bad news. *International Journal of Health Care Quality Assurance, 15*, 324–336.

Fallowfield, L., & Jenkins, V. (2004) Communicating sad, bad, and difficult news in medicine. *The Lancet, 363*, 312–319.

Glaser, B. G., & Strauss, A. L. (1968). *Time for dying.* New Brunswick, NJ: Aldine.

Gold, K. J. (2007). Navigating care after a baby dies: A systematic review of parent experiences with health providers. *Journal of Perinatology, 27*, 230–237.

Gyulay, J. (1989). Sudden death—No farewells. In The death of a child [Special issue]. *Issues In Comprehensive Pediatric Nursing, 12*, 71–102.

Hobgood, C. D., Tamayo-Sarver, J. H., Hollar, D. W., & Sawning, S. (2009). Grieving: Death notification skills and applications for fourth-year medical students. *Teaching & Learning In Medicine, 21*, 207–219.

Janzen, L., Cadell, S., & Westhues, A. (2003). From death notification through the funeral: Bereaved parents' experiences and their advice to professionals. *Omega: Journal of Death & Dying, 48*(2), 149–164.

Kirkley-Best, E., Kellner, K. R., & Ladue, T. (1984–1985). Attitudes toward stillbirth and death threat level in a sample of obstetricians. *Omega: Journal of Death and Dying, 15*, 317–327.

Leash, R. (1996). Death notification: Practical guidelines for health care professionals. *Critical Care Nursing Quarterly, 19*, 21–34.

Leon, I. G. (1992). Commentary: Providing versus packaging support for bereaved parents after perinatal loss. *Birth, 19*(2), 89–91.

Levetown, M. (2008). Communicating with children and families: From everyday interactions to skill in conveying distressing information. *Pediatrics, 121*, e1441–e1460.

MacDorman, M. F., & Kirmeyer, S. (2009). Fetal and perinatal mortality, United States, 2005. *National Vital Statistics, 57*, 1–19.

Mager, W. M., & Andrykowski, M. A. (2002). Communication in the cancer 'bad news' consultation: Patient perceptions and psychological adjustment. *Psycho-Oncology, 11*, 35–46.

Nordström, A. (2011). An exercise in death notification. *Medical Education, 45*, 1139–1140.

Peppers, L. G., & Knapp, R. J. (1980). Maternal reactions to involuntary fetal/infant death. *Psychiatry, 43155*–43159.

Ponce, A., Swor, R., Quest, T. E., Macy, M., Meurer, W., & Sasson, C. (2010). Death notification training for prehospital providers: A pilot study. *Prehospital Emergency Care, 14*, 537–542.

Prasad, V. (2010). Language in the end. *JGIM: Journal of General Internal Medicine, 25*(8), 884–885.

Ptacek, J. T., & Ellison, N. M. (2000). Health care providers' perspectives on breaking bad news to patients. *Critical Care Nursing, 23*(2), 51–59.

Pullen, S., & Nalos, D. (2009, February). *Giving birth to death: A quantitative study of patients' perceptions of the news delivery of stillbirth diagnosis by health care providers.* Paper presented at the meeting of the Western States Communication Association, Mesa, AZ.

Reddy, U. M. (2007). Prediction and prevention of recurrent stillbirth. *Obstetrics & Gynecology, 110*, 1151–1164.

Robson, S., Thompson, J., & Ellwood, D. (2006). Obstetric management of the next pregnancy after an unexplained stillbirth: An anonymous postal survey of Australian obstetricians. *Australian & New Zealand Journal of Obstetrics & Gynaecology, 46*, 278–281.

Säflund, K. (2003) *An analysis of parents' experiences and the caregivers' role following the birth of a stillborn child* (Unpublished doctoral dissertation). Karolinska Institutet Danderyds Sjukhus, Division of Obstetrics and Gynaecology, Stockholm, Sweden.

Säflund, K., Sjögren, B., & Wredling, R. (2002). Physicians' attitudes and advice concerning pregnancy subsequent to the birth of a stillborn child. *Journal of Psychosomatic Obstetrics & Gynecology, 23*, 109–115.

Säflund, K., Sjögren, B., & Wredling, R. (2004). The role of caregivers after a stillbirth: Views and experiences of parents. *Birth, 31*, 132–137.

Salander, P. (2002). Bad news from the patient's perspective: An analysis of the written narratives of newly diagnosed cancer patients. *Social Science & Medicine, 55*, 721–732.

Schott, J., Henley, A., & Kohner, N. (2007). *Pregnancy loss and the death of a baby: Guidelines for professionals* (3rd ed.). Shepperton on Thames, United Kingdom: Bosun Press.

Smith-Cumberland, T. (2006). The evaluation of two death education programs for EMTs using the theory of planned behavior. *Death Studies, 30,* 637–647.

Smith-Cumberland, T., & Feldman, R. (2006). EMT's attitudes toward death before and after a death education program. *Prehospital Emergency Care, 10*(1), 89–95.

Statham, H., & Dimavicius, J. (1992). Commentary: How do you give the bad news to parents? *Birth, 19,* 103–104.

Stewart, A. E., Lord, J. H., & Mercer, D. L. (2000). A survey of professionals' training and experiences in delivering death notifications. *Death Studies, 24,* 611–631.

Strauss, A., & Corbin, J. M. (1990). *Basics of qualitative research: Grounded theory procedures and techniques.* Thousand Oaks, CA: Sage.

Strauss, R. P., Sharp, M. C., Lorch, C., & Kachalia, B. (1995). Physicians and the communication of "bad news": Parent experiences of being informed of their child's cleft lip and/or palate. *Pediatrics, 96,* 82–89.

Trulsson, O., & Radestad, I. (2004). The silent child—Mothers' experiences before, during, and after stillbirth. *Birth, 31,* 189–195.

Villagran, M., Goldsmith, J., Wittenberg-Lyles, E. M., & Baldwin, P. (2010). Creating COMFORT: A communication-based model for breaking bad news. *Communication Education, 59,* 220–234.

Watson, B., & Gallois, C. (1998). Nurturing communication by health professionals toward patients: A communication accommodation theory approach. *Health Communication, 10,* 343–355.

Widger, K., & Picot, C. (2008). Parents' perceptions of the quality of pediatric and perinatal end-of-life care. *Pediatric Nursing, 34,* 53–58.

Yardley, S. J., Davis, C. L., & Sheldon, F. (2001). Receiving a diagnosis of lung cancer: Patients' interpretations, perceptions and perspectives. *Palliative Medicine, 15,* 379–386.

APPENDIX 1: Key Distinctions Between Parent Groups

	Parents reporting positive perceptions	Parents reporting negative perceptions
Core stillbirth notification experience (differing in form and frequency between groups)	Delay of news delivery Expression of sympathy • paired with intensifiers • nonverbal expressions of sympathy Communication of death • nonverbal coupled with verbal notification	Delay of news delivery • topic avoidance by HCP Expression of sympathy • simple statements Communication of death • implied statements of death
Shared experiences in stillbirth notification (differing in focus and timing between groups)	Communication re: options • options offered or limits on options explained Expressed uncertainty • expressed uncertainty about how to deliver news • uncertainty paired with hopefulness • HCP gave, or desired to find, cause of death Noted exit of HCP • HCP presence after news delivery	Communication re: options • options limited without explanation Expressed uncertainty • expressed uncertainty re: baby's condition or how to perform exam • uncertainty paired with hopelessness Noted exit of HCP • immediate HCP exit
Opposing experiences in stillbirth notification	Support of parent emotion Information provision Continuity of care	Suppression of parent emotion Lack of information provision Lack of continuity of care

Informing Social Work Practice Through Research With Parent Caregivers of a Child With a Life-Limiting Illness

SUSAN CADELL

School of Social Work, Renison University College, University of Waterloo, Waterloo, Ontario, Canada

KIMBERLY KENNEDY

Faculty of Social Work, Wilfrid Laurier University, Kitchener, Ontario, Canada

DAVID HEMSWORTH

Faculty of Applied & Professional Studies, School of Business & Economics, Nipissing University, North Bay, Ontario, Canada

Pediatric palliative care is an evolving field of practice in social work. As such, research plays a critical role in informing best social work practices in this area. For parents, caring for a child with a life-limiting illness (LLI) is a stressful experience that compounds the usual challenges of parenting. The negative aspects of caring for a child with an LLI are well documented. In the face of such adversity, parent caregivers can also experience positive changes caring for children with even the most serious conditions. This article presents results from a research study of posttraumatic growth in parents who are caring for a child with a LLI. Using mixed methods, two overarching themes were prominent in both the quantitative and qualitative data. The first describes stress related to financial burden associated with caregiving. The second theme concerns the posttraumatic growth experienced by the parent caregivers. The quantitative and qualitative data have been woven together to underscore issues and parental perspectives related to these two themes. This provides a unique and important platform for parent

---

This work was supported by Canadian Institutes of Health Research Grants PET–69769 and MOP–79526.

caregivers' experiences that can inform the work of social workers and other pediatric palliative care professionals.

Pediatric palliative care (PPC) is an evolving field of practice in social work, yet few health care professionals are educated specifically in PPC (Benini, Spizzichino, Trapanotto, & Ferrante, 2008; Gilmer, Foster, Bell, Mulder, & Carter, 2012; Liben, Papadatou, & Wolfe, 2008) and few social workers receive more than on-the-job training (Jones, 2005), highlighting the need for the examination of best practices. In addition, more research is needed in the area of pediatric palliative care that will inform practice (Davies et al., 2011; Kumar, 2011), especially for social workers.

For parents, caring for a child within the context of PPC is a stressful experience that compounds the usual challenges of parenting. The negative aspects of caring for a child with a life-limiting illness (LLI) are well-documented (Contro, Larson, Scofield, Sourkes & Cohen, 2002; Rapoport, Beaune, Weingarten, Rugg, & Newman, 2012; Steele, 2000; Steele & Davies, 2006). From a clinical perspective, parent caregivers are also seen to undergo positive changes within themselves and their relationships. Yet we know little about the experience of personal growth in people who care for others. This article presents selected results from a mixed-methods research study of posttraumatic growth in parents who are caring for a child with a LLI. The question that drove this research investigation was "What are the factors that allow parents who are caring for a child with a life-limiting illness to survive and even grow in the face of adversity?"

CHILDREN WITH LLIs AND THEIR PARENT CAREGIVERS

The context for this study is parents whose children have a LLI and are not expected to live into full adulthood. Pediatric palliative care differs from adult care in that it often begins earlier and lasts longer: It is not care only at the end of life. The Association for Children with Life-Threatening or Terminal Conditions and Their Families and the Royal College of Paediatrics and Child Health in the United Kingdom recognized four distinct categories of disease conditions cared for in PPC (ACT/RCPHC, 2003). The conditions that affect children are physiologically diverse and contribute to varied life expectancies (Ashby, Kosky, Laver, & Sims, 1991; Davies & Howell, 1998; Goldman, 1996)— such as cancer, neuromuscular diseases, neurodegenerative diseases, metabolic disorders, genetic syndromes, and cellular diseases. These conditions are all potentially LLIs yet they have diverse trajectories and time courses.

Regardless of diagnosis or prognosis, parents are central to the care that children with LLIs receive, both at home and in health care settings. The experience of caregiving varies greatly from family to family and diagnosis to diagnosis. Being the parent of a child with a condition that has the possibility of either cure or death carries with it a significant burden. Opportunities for treatments and interventions that may result in a cure may contribute to uncertainty about the child's future, including long-term health (Bluebond-Langner, Belasco, Goldman, & Belasco, 2007). Children and youth who require intensive medical therapy and management over a prolonged period of time, without any known chance of cure, may rely heavily on their parents. Parental caregiving for these children can be a very involved process, with losses of significant milestones occurring throughout the illness trajectory. The role of the parent caregiver is continually changing. Whether a child's disease requires invasive treatments to cure or constant monitoring and management over time, dependency on parents is likely to increase, either temporarily or permanently. For example, if a child's energy level or mobility declines, he or she may eventually be forced to rely on parents for all personal care needs. Several conditions can render children completely dependent on their parents for communication, feeding, and mobility. These children often require a complex care plan with parents providing constant care over extended periods of time. Families often make significant adjustments in their lives that have broader effects and touch every member of the family. Employment may change for one or both parents, adding to family stress. Parents must navigate the various systems involved in the care of their child, interfacing with multiple specialists and advocating for resources. In a field where prognostic predictions can be poor and nothing is guaranteed, parents face the ongoing ambiguity about the future health, wellness, and functioning of their child.

THEORETICAL FRAMEWORK

This research is informed by the theoretical framework of stress and coping, as proposed by Folkman (1997), and the construct of posttraumatic growth, as elaborated by Tedeschi and Calhoun (Tedeschi & Calhoun, 1996; Tedeschi, Park, & Calhoun, 1998). The original model of transactional coping proposed by Lazarus and Folkman (1984) included positive emotion as a possible outcome only when there was a favorable resolution to a threatening event. Folkman (1997) reworked the original model, introducing the possibility of experiencing positive emotions when there is not a favorable resolution or no resolution at all. The revised model is designed to indicate that positive emotions occur through a process of meaning making and that positive and negative psychological states coexist. A feedback loop that was inserted into the revised model acknowledges that distress continues despite the positive aspects. A similar feedback loop of wisdom and distress also occurs in Tedeschi and Calhoun's (1996) conceptualization of posttraumatic growth.

Consensus exists among researchers about aspects of personal growth—including the experience of new possibilities, enhanced relationships, enhanced strength, increased appreciation of life, and spiritual change (McMillen & Fisher, 1998; Tedeschi & Calhoun, 1995). The occurrence of personal growth after adversity is referred to by various names—including posttraumatic growth (Tedeschi & Calhoun, 1995; Tedeschi et al., 1998), stress-related growth (Park, Cohen, & Murch, 1996), positive by-products (McMillen & Cook, 2003), and thriving (Ickovics & Park, 1998). Posttraumatic growth refers to the positive changes that people experience as a result of adverse circumstances (Joseph & Linley, 2008; McMillen, 1999; Park, Cohen & Murch, 1996; Tedeschi et al., 1998). Resilience is defined as the ability to adapt to, cope with, and even be strengthened by adverse circumstances (Begun, 1993; Masten, Best, & Garmezy, 1990, 1994; Scannapieco & Jackson, 1996). Growth goes beyond resilience in that it encompasses thriving—a gain that surpasses a return to the prestressful state (Ickovics & Park, 1998). People have been observed to experience benefit in struggling with threatening experiences as diverse as natural disasters (Thompson, 1985), war (Aldwin, Levenson, & Spiro, 1994; Elder & Clipp, 1989), disability (Dunn, 1994; McMillen & Cook, 2003), rape (Burt & Katz, 1987), cancer (Barakat, Alderfer, & Kazak, 2006; Thornton & Perez, 2006), bereavement (Calhoun & Tedeschi, 1990; Frantz, Trolley, & Farrell, 1998; Kessler, 1987; Lehman et al., 1993), and recovery from chemical dependency (McMillen, Howard, Nower, & Chung, 2001).

METHODS

Participant Selection and Procedures

This mixed-methods study was approved ethically in all institutions in which members of the research team were located: in total, four universities and six clinical sites. Recruitment occurred through various methods as suited the individual institutions. In some places, posters were visible asking if parents were caring for a child with a LLI and interested in participation in the project. Some organizations made the poster or information available on their website, others sent letters. Recruitment took place in the United States and Canada and questionnaires were available in both English and French (the official languages of Canada). Parents were included if they were currently caring for a child with a LLI aged 19 or younger. The posters, letters, and all information about the study directed parents to a toll-free number. Having the parents contact the research office directly guaranteed the participants confidentiality in relation to the referring institution. Information about source of referral was not collected so an analysis could not be conducted regarding any difference this may have made. More than one caregiver could participate for each child. In addition to parents, grandparents, foster parents, and stepparents participated if they were directly involved in caring for a child with a LLI.

The study was mixed methods in two phases. The first phase used quantitative methods and consisted of a questionnaire measuring personal resources, spirituality, stress, and personal growth for parents caring for a child with a LLI. When parents left a phone message, their call was returned, the study was explained to them and if they agreed to participate, a questionnaire package was mailed to them. The package included an information letter, a stamped addressed return envelope, and $20 for their participation.

The questionnaire package was designed to take parents approximately 30 to 90 minutes to complete. The packages were mailed rather than attempting to administer the questionnaires by phone so that the parents could fill them in at their own pace. While this potentially has methodological implications, it was determined to be the least intrusive approach for these parents who are actively caring for seriously ill children. Reminder notices were sent to participants who did not return the questionnaire after approximately 45 days. Participants were assured that all information collected would be kept strictly confidential. Identification numbers were used on written forms and all identifying information was locked up and/or password protected. All procedures were in accordance with the ethics guidelines at the home institution. Overall, 367 people called for information about the study. Three hundred and forty packages were mailed out (12 did not qualify because of the child's age, type of illness, or the child was deceased; 5 were not interested; and 10 could not be reached). In total, 273 completed questionnaires were returned.

The second phase of the research consisted of semi-structured interviews. Parents who filled in the questionnaire and agreed to be contacted for follow-up were grouped according to their scores on the Posttraumatic Growth Inventory (Tedeschi & Calhoun, 1996). Beginning with the highest and the lowest scores, parents who were located in areas that were geographically accessible were invited to participate in interviews. In total, 23 individuals were interviewed in either Canada or the United States. Of the thirty-six couples who completed surveys, 12 were interviewed together. The couple interviews aimed to promote an understanding of how posttraumatic growth occurs and is sustained in couples. All couples were living in Canada. The full number of individual and couple interviews was 35 (47 people participating).

Research trainees who worked with the principal investigator or a member of the research team conducted the participant interviews. A semi-structured interview schedule guided the interviews and participants were given a check for $30 to thank them for their time and participation. Questions addressed the areas identified as possible factors in growth. Participants were also asked if there were aspects of their experience that they considered beneficial to them that may not have been covered by the questionnaires. Interviews were audiotaped with the participant's consent. All research trainees had completed at least the first year of a Master's of social science program involving course work in interviewing skills, practice opportunities, and the completion of a 6-month clinical placement. Additional training included instruction of how to interview regarding sensitive topics and self-care. If the interviewer deemed the participant to be in distress throughout or following the interview, information was provided regarding sources of immediate support in their community.

Instruments

The questionnaire in the first phase was comporised of eight instruments overall. In addition to those described below, six other measures were used that are not reported on here. They included measures of self-esteem, spirituality, optimism, burden, meaning in caregiving, and depression. The full set of instruments, the model, and the hypotheses can be found in Schneider, Steele, Cadell, and Hemsworth (2011).

DEMOGRAPHICS

The instrument was designed to collect demographic and illness-related information from family caregivers of older adults and was adapted for parents. The instrument included a series of questions about length of time since the child had been diagnosed and how long the participant had been providing care.

POSTTRAUMATIC GROWTH

The variable of growth was measured using five subscales of the Posttraumatic Growth Inventory (PTGI). The PTGI was developed to measure positive outcomes of trauma and has 21 items which are answered with a 6-point Likert scale (Tedeschi & Calhoun, 1996). The PTGI was chosen for this study because its subscales represent the commonalities of personal growth, even though caregiving is not generally represented as traumatic. Respondents of the PTGI are asked to rate statements about changes in their lives as a result of their crisis (Tedeschi & Calhoun, 1996). For the purpose of this research, the word "crisis" was replaced with "caregiving" in order to tailor the questionnaire wording to the population for which it is intended (Cadell & Sullivan, 2006). The PTGI measures five factors: *new possibilities*, *relating to others*, *personal strength*, *appreciation of life*, and *spiritual change*. The scale was tested on 604 undergraduate students in the United States. An alpha coefficient of .90 was reported with test-retest reliability at .71 over 2 months.

For the second phase, an interview guide was developed that asked questions based on the aforementioned instruments. The research team developed the interview guide based in part on prior interviews about post-traumatic growth in a different population (Cadell, 2007). Consultation with a parent advisory panel also took place.

Data Analysis

In the quantitative phase, data were entered into Microsoft Excel 2003 for preprocessing, data cleaning, reversal of items, and determination of scale composites. Missing data was dealt with using pairwise deletion, rather than mean substitution; the average of remaining reported values was used to replace missing scale items. IBM SPSS Version 19 (IBM Corp., Armonk, NY, USA) was then used for the statistical analyses. Descriptive statistics were run, as appropriate. For example, frequencies and percentage for categorical variables and means were generated, while standard deviations for continuous variables and Pearson correlations, as appropriate for level of variable, were performed. All tests were two-tailed, and the level of significance was set at .05, so p values greater than .05 were reported as statistically significant.

In the second phase, content analyses were performed by reviewing the transcripts of the interviews for the purposes of this article. The research plan includes structural equation modeling of the first phase data and a full grounded theory analysis of the qualitative data which will be reported in subsequent articles.

RESULTS

Sample Description

Two hundred seventy-three caregivers answered the questionnaire in the first phase, of whom, 128 (47%) were from Canada and 145 (53%) were from the United States. The sample included 216 mothers, 49 fathers, and 8 grandmothers. Twenty-three parents were caring for more than one child with a LLI and there were 35 mother/father couples and 3 parent/grandparent respondents. Information was not tracked about foster and stepparents, but we know from interviews that a number of caregivers were related in this manner. The average age of the caregivers was 41.74 years ($SD = 7.61$) and 80.2% were married (see Table 1 for additional demographics).

Two hundred and thirty-five children, ranging in age from 6 months to 20 years, were being cared for in the study. The duration of years spent caring ranged from less than 1 to over 19 years. No difference in PTGI scores was found in relation to time caregiving or years since diagnosis. A similar lack of relationship between time and growth was found in HIV carers

TABLE 1 Description of Participants

Variable	Means	
	M (*SD*)	Range
Age in years	41.74 (7.61)	22.99–68.38
Hours per week spent caregiving	62.16 (44.72)	0–126
	Frequencies (*n* = 273)	
	Count	Percent
Gender		
Female	224	82.1
Male	49	17.9
Marital status		
Married	219	80.2
Never married	13	4.8
Divorced/Widowed	36	13.2
Other/did not answer	5	1.8
Relation to child		
Mother	216	79.1
Father	49	17.9
Grandmother	8	2.9
Size of community		
Metropolitan area/large city	120	44.0
Medium city/small city	91	33.3
Smaller communities	62	22.7
Average household income per year ($)		
<40,000	60	22.8
40,000–79,999	86	32.6
80,000–119,000	70	26.5
>120,000	48	18.1
Income changed after child's illness		
No	96	35.3
Yes	176	64.7
Current income meets needs		
Totally inadequate	10	3.7
Not very well	30	11.1
With some difficulty	77	28.4
Adequately	99	36.5
Very well	36	13.3
Completely	19	7.0
Highest level of education		
Less than high school	13	4.8
Completed high school	98	36.2
Postsecondary education	160	58.0

Note. Numbers do not always add up to 273 because of missing data.

(Cadell, Regehr, & Hemsworth, 2003; Cadell & Sullivan, 2006). A varied spectrum of pediatric illnesses were represented; diagnoses represented each of the four recognized quadrants of disease conditions of children cared for in PPC (see Table 2; Anonymous, 1997). The return rate for the questionnaires was 82.6%; with 94% of these caregivers consenting to be contacted about follow-up research.

Thematic Findings

The results presented two overarching themes that were prominent in both the quantitative and qualitative data. The first theme described stress related to financial burden associated with caregiving. Although it is acknowledged that stressors are certainly not limited to the economic when caring for a child with a LLI, this was an area of trepidation shared by many families. The second theme concerns the posttraumatic growth experienced by the parent caregivers. The quantitative and qualitative data has been woven together to underscore issues and parental perspectives related to these two themes. The names and other identifying information have been changed to maintain confidentiality of participants.

Financial Stress Associated With Caregiving

As seen in Table 1, the majority of parent caregivers (58%) had acquired some level of post-secondary education with many (45%) reporting household incomes of $80,000 a year or greater. Approximately 43% of participants reported that they had at least some difficulty meeting needs within their current income. This was more than double the number of parents who

TABLE 2 Children's Diagnoses by Quadrant

Quadrant	Description	Count	Percent
1	Life-threatening conditions for which curative treatment may be feasible but can fail (e.g., cancer, irreversible organ failures).	30	11.1
2	Conditions where premature death is inevitable, but with long periods of intensive treatment aimed at prolonging life and allowing participation in normal activities (e.g., cystic fibrosis).	185	68.5
3	Progressive conditions without curative treatment options, where treatment is exclusively palliative and may extend over many years (e.g., neurodegenerative, metabolic disease).	26	9.6
4	Irreversible but nonprogressive conditions with severe disability susceptible to health complications and premature death (e.g., anoxic brain injury, severe cerebral palsy).	29	10.7
Total		270	100

Note. Three families did not provide information about their child's diagnosis. Quadrant descriptions (Anonymous, 1997).

responded that they were able to meet needs *very well* or *completely*. The financial struggles that families were confronted with were not solely related to their income. Even those with higher average incomes spoke of being challenged financially as expenses accumulated over time. One mother of a 2-year-old girl commented:

> Everything is based on income, not based on how much money you actually have. They might take at least half of it. Sometimes it's frustrating because our income might be higher than some other people, but that doesn't mean we're not needing it more … , like they don't take into consideration oh they're paying $500 a month in homecare and $200 a month for her feed, and you know, they make all this money they should be able to do without it.

Caregivers spoke of the burden of major expenses such as costly renovations, having to buy a reliable vehicle to get a child to appointments, or moving to a different part of the province to be closer to the hospital. The seemingly minor expenses—such as travel to and from the hospital, parking, meals, and basic supplies like diapers—were also reported to contribute to the financial stress of families. A mother recounted her family's story:

> We've had to refinance our home because of debt that was incurred because of going back and forth [to the hospital], and still having to go back and forth, you know, we're still having to rack up our credit cards again—sometimes extra costs, like the feeding, homecare, financial things. We'd like to expand our house, but with all the extra responsibility financially, well right now she's small it's not such a big deal, but as she grows … bigger challenges.

Financial barriers prevented caregivers from accessing essential training, supports, and resources. The stepfather of a 7-year-old son clarified that it is not just the child that loses out when programs are not funded—it is the entire family:

> So, just talking about [my wife] taking immersion sign language courses, we can't get funding for that and that's for us to learn to communicate with [our son]! And like that's a two–three thousand dollar bill out of your pocket for a week, you know? And if you can't get financing for respite and for programs that's out of your pocket. You have your travel, that's out of your pocket. You have to pay for the course, that's out of your pocket—your hotel, your meals, everything, and to—for him to benefit! Like that's—I don't know if it's right, I don't know if it's wrong, but I think we feel as a family there should be more support for stuff like that because it—he's not suffering, it's the entire family having to deal with this, you know?

Sixty-five percent of caregivers reported that their family income changed due to their child's illness. Almost one-half (49%) of the parents reported a change in their employment status as a result of their caregiving role, the vast majority of whom were mothers (see Table 3). For many, the decision to continue working full-time or stay at home to care for their child did not come easily. The mother of a 17-year-old daughter shared:

> I have my family behind me, you know, like telling me you have to be home, "that's where you're needed right now," and "you shouldn't be working." But then, I know that I have to work. It's not possible financially if I stop working, but at the same time you get to wonder, I don't know .... We're just at the point right now if I don't work it's going to go very bad.

TABLE 3 Comparison of Female and Male Participants

Variable	M (SD)	
	Women	Men
Age in years	41.19 (7.62)	44.29 (7.08)
Hours per week spent caregiving	68.0 (43.88)	37.64 (39.97)
	Frequencies (n = 273)			
	Count		Percent	
	Women	Men	Women	Men
Employment status				
Full time	70	44	31.3	89.8
Part time	37	1	16.5	2.0
Paid leave	5	0	2.2	0
Unpaid leave	3	0	1.3	0
Self-employed	13	3	5.8	6.1
Not employed	78	0	34.8	0
Other	18	1	8.0	2.0
Change in employment status				
No	94	42	43.1	85.7
Yes	124	7	56.9	14.3
Highest level of education				
High school or less	35	5	15.6	10.2
Some postsecondary	59	12	26.3	24.5
College diploma	30	9	13.4	18.4
Undergraduate degree	51	13	22.8	26.5
Postgraduate degree	47	10	21.0	20.4
Other (not specified)	2	0	0.9	0
Total participants	224	49	82.1	17.9

Note. Numbers do not always add up to 273 because of missing data.

Parents reported turning down promotions at work that would have meant more money, but less time to fulfill caregiving responsibilities. The adoptive father of a 12-year-old son shared:

> [My wife] could have been promoted and so could have I, but we kind of stayed in jobs that were somewhat—we can work from home on some days. We don't really have any staff we have to manage, if you know what I mean. ... We could have probably moved to somewhere and moved up, but we just kind of—I limited myself to say I won't drive more than 45 minutes ... . So I haven't taken certain jobs.

Parents cited lack of reliable homecare, in-home support, and respite services as common reasons for choosing to leave the workplace to care for their child full-time. A consistent theme heard during the caregiver interviews was the stress and frustration associated with securing reliable professional care for their child. One mother of a 6-year-old daughter commented: "And the homecare was just a disaster. I was more stressed with homecare then I was with (our daughter)."

Another parent of a 7-year-old son related:

> Trying to get adequate staffing for him—we've had one or two girls that were more of a nightmare than anything else and one girl was actually working out good, but she couldn't handle (our son) because he's high-maintenance and she just phoned one day and said, "I'm quitting." So, I said, "Oh, so this is 2 weeks' notice? That's fine." "No, I'm just not coming in."

Parents spent substantial amounts of time searching for eligible funding subsidies, grants, and tax credits related to their child. Many recounted how time consuming it had been to find relevant services, supports, and resources for their children. Some mothers relinquished full-time positions in order to have more time to search and follow up on information that would benefit their family. One mother stated:

> Lucky enough when I was working full-time during my lunch I would spend my whole entire lunch hour doing things on my desk. Searching things—and that really helped me out during that time ... . Just going through and typing things going to another link back and forth back and forth. So! But you know not everyone has time to do that depending on how sick your child is, too. What happens to them when they come out of the hospital?

Resource and funding information was often discovered through other parent caregivers, with some families going for years before learning about beneficial programs. Mothers and fathers expressed their displeasure and frustrations with the lack of information sharing that took place by professionals. One caregiver stated:

> Oh, the system's gotta be a little more open for parents, families to help them find more resources—to actually have people stand up and say, "Hey you! We've got something for you," rather than as a family having to actually track this stuff down because that's a big freakin' headache trying to track down services for your children. I can't think of anything that's any worse than that throughout this whole process.

Posttraumatic Growth

All participants answered questions about the growth they experienced in relation to their child's illness using the Posttraumatic Growth Inventory (Tedeschi & Calhoun, 1996). The mean of the overall PTGI score for these caregivers is 62.9 (with a standard deviation of 20.8) out of a possible 126. The scores on the subscales can be found in Table 4. There is no established cutoff for posttraumatic growth, but this score puts the mean of these parents in the high end of the range of experiencing the changes to a *small* degree (more than *very small* but less than *moderate*).

All aspects of posttraumatic growth (experiencing new possibilities, enhanced relationships, enhanced strength, increased appreciation of life, and spiritual change) came out in the interviews with caregivers. There were four subthemes that emerged in more detail and have been highlighted here: growth alongside distress, building connections, becoming an advocate, and growth through self-care.

Growth Alongside Distress

> And so we're always kind of day-by-day ... having the experience of not knowing if he's going to live to see his next birthday, but grooming him for adulthood ... so it's kind of interesting. It's like half of my day is filled with elation and half of it is grief. It's a constant grieving process. But it's also really thrilling and exciting.

These words, shared by the mother of her 9-year-old son, captured the nature of the growth that was expressed by caregiving parents. It is tinged

TABLE 4 Means and Standard Deviations for PTGI Scales ($N = 273$)

	Total PTGI	Relationships with others	New possibilities	Personal strength	Spiritual change	Appreciation of life
M	62.94	20.58	13.72	13.16	4.68	10.80
SD	20.80	7.31	6.30	4.82	3.53	3.42

Note. PTGI = Posttraumatic Growth Inventory.

with ongoing stress. A father of a 15-year-old expressed the process of coming to truly appreciate his daughter for who she was, rather than letting her illness identify her:

> A real significant thing was me realizing at one point how amazing [my daughter] was. ... in some ways it took a really long time to trust her to know what was best for herself. I think that's been the cool thing is realizing she's just a kid. And um, and I think because of that we've kind of stopped seeing her muscle disease, we just see her.

Some parents made a connection between the challenges they have faced as caregivers and positive changes they have experienced. Making meaning of the child's illness and the caregiving experience brought growth to some. One father of an 8-year-old commented:

> But, I believe there's a spirit, something very strong and their message is all about loving each other and trying to find the big picture and when I heard about [my son's condition], that night, often I do a prayer, I was cursing [that spirit]—but like, why, if you're love, why do this? And I got it. I got ... he is still the same, he's still [my son], he's full of life, and that nice smile of his, and the gap between his teeth because he knocked his tooth loose. It was just so cute. That's why. He can take it, he's strong-willed. There's a reason for everything.

The father of a 12-year-old boy shared:

> I felt like my struggle was just part of my becoming a better person, like a more Godly person, or a more God-centered person and that God has a, you know, wants me to help others in that same .... Because what we found, very soon after we started going to support groups, we learned that even though we're all strangers in the room, we all sought a deeper understanding having all gone through the same experiences.

The comment of this father exemplified how all five concepts of growth can be interconnected. He spoke of personal strength, spiritual connection, supporting relationships with others, new opportunities, and taking a different perspective on life.

Building Connections

The message that only those who have a child with a LLI can begin to understand what this experience is like was expressed in almost every caregiver interview. It was communicated that not only friends and colleagues have difficulty grasping the finality of a child having an illness that will be "forever," family members also struggled with the idea. It was important for many caregivers to connect with people facing similar circumstances. Personal connections were made through organization(s) dedicated to their child's disease, by attending conferences, and meeting families in formal and informal settings such as hospitals, clinics, and hospices. A couple with a 9-year-old daughter clarified the value of these connections:

> Dad: They don't—they'll never understand. They think it's something that's going to be cured like in a month or two, a year, and it's gonna be over.

> Mom: No matter how many times you say it—that's why going to the (MPS) conference, it's like—ahhhh—I'm like, you don't have to explain anything, all these parents know it all. It's like a family.

Caregivers felt that connections with others did not have to be through face to face contact to be valued. Many connected with other parents through Internet sites and blogs. "Talking" with other caregiving parents not only served as a reminder that they were not alone, but a number of parents used this venue to post questions and get advice on such issues as medical procedures and treatment options. Parents reported using the experiences of others to evaluate their child's options, guide decisions, and set realistic expectations. One mother of a 6-year-old girl described her online communication as her "lifeline." She elaborated:

> Everything I've learnt I have learnt through there (Internet) ... if ever I needed any information I go on to it and ask and you get lots of answers back. Most the same answers, but some different and it's just been the best thing for me ... . Like it's, you know, it's so sad to say it, but it's nice to have somebody else that knows exactly what you're going through.

Becoming an Advocate

Becoming an advocate was one skill that caregivers reported discovering in themselves. As a response to the perceived lack of understanding about pediatric LLI, parents spoke of their families becoming involved in campaigns to raise awareness in their home communities. Public speaking and organizing community events were additional strengths realized by parents through the process of caregiving. One mother, who described herself as the quiet kid, who "never used to really ask for anything," organized a walk to raise awareness and educate neighbors about her daughter's disease. She contacted radio stations and newspapers to share her story. Displaying courage that seemed to surprise her more than anyone, she travelled to Ottawa with her local member of parliament to meet with the federal minister of health about her daughter getting access to a medication not available in Canada.

> I kept searching on the Internet and found the Canadian [rare disease] Society; called them, talked to the lady that was in charge and she said, "Yeah, you know what, you have to fight real hard." ... (We) called the radio stations, newspapers and—our daughter needed a medication to slow down the progress of this disease—we started a walk that year too to raise awareness and even our MP (Member of Parliament) did the walk! So he came to the walk, our pharmacist at the drug store came to the walk, and the geneticist came to the walk, so they had a little pow-wow.

Other caregivers spoke of advocating not only for their child and family, but for those they felt were not in a position to fight for their rights. The sense of injustice seemed to be the catalyst for parents to take action, or as one mother described it "raising a big stink."

> The complexity of the support system.... It was ridiculous and now I ended up actually writing a letter to the minister and raising a big stink about it because I don't—I'm pretty stubborn and I was having trouble getting stuff—it took us 11 months to get a bath chair, which is pretty crucial and I was thinking, I've got a friend in town with a boy who's got mito who's a single mom, on welfare, can't work, she's sick, no support, she can't do that. She can't spend 3 days a week fighting with her worker to try and get something done. And once I started making a stink about it some changes happened, things started happening quicker. I'm hoping it's happening quicker for everybody and not just me because I'm annoying.

For other parent caregivers, the battles were less about wanting to change the system or the views of others, and more about ensuring their child was getting the best care possible—whatever it took: "That's what you do and what you've got to do and that's what we do. Keep fighting—pick your battles and chase 'em."

Growth Through Self-Care

An area of growth shared by parents was learning to acknowledge their personal needs and the importance of self-care; although, practicing self-care was not always a luxury caregivers felt they had time to afford themselves on a regular basis. Self-care practices for some caregivers were about revitalization; for example, going to the gym or devoting time to themselves. However, there were reports of self-care rituals that were more closely associated with various aspect of growth for different caregivers. For example, appreciating and nurturing relationships in environments where their family was not judged or viewed as different.

Reports of self-care included seeking professional support. A handful of caregivers talked about taking part in individual or couples counseling. The mother of a 12-year-old boy spoke of moving toward acceptance after seeking assistance from a social worker:

> So, I went through our work. So, I went through those questions with [my social worker] .... She was awesome because I just was able to sit and talk and she just asked questions that she—well, they needed to be asked. And I just worked through it.

Self-identification of physical and emotional concerns appeared to be key to the well-being of caregivers. While many parents praised the support they received from health care providers, others felt they showed little consideration for their well-being. This oversight was especially relevant for mothers who, in most cases, were fulfilling the bulk of the manual caregiving within the family—including lifting, bathing, toileting and caring out therapy routines. One mother of a 17-year-old girl, with limited mobility, stated:

> I hurt my back, I hurt my shoulder ... and then (my physiotherapist) gave me that book that shows you how to transfer people. Nobody ever told me that! Like where's the class for the mom or the dad or anybody taking care of those people. Why is it that we're not offered to go to class like that?

Caregiving parents noted that their ability to cope emotionally with the demands of caregiving was at times disregarded by health care providers. The same mother stated, "I don't understand why they treat my daughter, but don't ask me, you know, do you have what it takes?" Others shared their impression that certain members of the health care team seemed to intentionally ignore or avoid parents, lest they seek support for personal or relationship concerns. A foster mother of a 9-year-old boy advised:

> I think [health care professionals] need to be asking how are we coping— are we doing okay, do we need any help with anything? ... Just—I mean, it sounds so trivial and so small, but for sometimes it's—and when he was in the hospital, like wandering through the hallways and stuff at night time, like nobody ever asked, "Are you okay?" or anything like that.

It was noted that emotional support was not only lacking for parents at times but for healthy siblings as well. The mother of a 17-year-old added: "One thing I should have mentioned and I haven't, is the support for the siblings .... I mean, there's no support out there for the siblings."

DISCUSSION

The 235 children being cared for by participants of the study had a wide variety of illnesses that corresponded to the categories recognized by the

Association for Children with Life Threatening or Terminal Conditions and Their Families and the Royal College of Paediatrics and Child Health in PPC (Anonymous, 1997; see Table 2). Thus, we established a cohort that paralleled the broad experiences of families engaged in pediatric palliative care. The caregivers in the first phase included 36 couples where both parents filled in questionnaires concerning their individual experiences of caring for a child with a LLI—a noteworthy result as few fathers participate in research concerning pediatric palliative care (Macdonald, Chilibeck, Affleck, & Cadell, 2010) and their experiences are known to be different from mothers' (Davies et al., 2004). No known research has examined couples caring together. Differences in the overall sample based on gender were reported on in Schneider et al. (2011).

The themes of financial stress associated with caregiving and personal growth were central issues for parents, as was established through quantitative reports and during the interviews that followed. Having interwoven the quantitative and qualitative data related to these themes, this report more thoroughly demonstrates the nuances associated with financial matters and posttraumatic growth. The relationship between the positives and negatives experienced by families would not necessarily be evident through examination of the quantitative data alone.

Financial Stress Associated With Caregiving

Parent caregivers living in both Canada and the United States expressed financial stresses even with the presence of universal health care in Canada. Despite high levels of education and reasonably high household incomes, more than twice as many caregivers endorsed having at least some difficulty meeting needs with their current income compared to those who had no difficulty. Finances were affected by the monetary costs, as well as the time required to carry out duties associated with caregiving—such as accompanying children to appointments, attending meetings, and searching for resources and supports. This was consistent with earlier findings that families often face financial instability as a consequence of added medical and equipment expenses, child care, travel to and from hospital, and time away from work (Corden, Sloper, & Sainsbury, 2002; Monterosso, Kristjanson, Aoun, & Phillips, 2007; Morrod, 2004; Parker, 1996). In addition, to the accumulation of smaller expenses, parents spoke of costly renovations to their homes, having to buy new vehicles, and relocating their family closer to the hospital where their ill child was receiving care.

Approximately one-half of the caregiving parents (49%) underwent changes in their employment status as a result of their caregiving role. As reported in Schneider et al. (2011), it was generally women who experienced these changes (see Table 3). Exploring whether the changes were voluntary and the disproportionate effect on women's employment status will be an important area for future research. Parents in the current study expressed the stress and frustration associated with finding and securing programs and resources, in particular reliable homecare, in-home supports, and respite services. Lack of dependable care and the demands of caregiving led some to decrease the number of hours they worked, turn down promotions, or to leave the workplace completely in order to care for their child full-time.

There was a strong sense from the parent caregivers that there is a lack of understanding of the overall costs associated with caring for a child with a LLI. This oversight included health care professionals who unwittingly added to the financial burden. Social workers should consider the practices of their organization to determine how they may be adding to the expenses accrued by families. Coordinating clinic visits to decrease travel to and from hospitals, extending clinic hours one evening a month so parents do not have to take time off from work, providing child care, meal vouchers, and free parking to families are strategizes to help mitigate costs. Systemic changes to help ease the cost of care include opening satellite offices, partnering with care agencies in the communities where families are living, and changing illegibility criteria and time lines for government programs, such the compassionate care benefits.

Parent caregivers expressed disappointment over having gone for extended periods of time before learning about beneficial programs, including funding opportunities. They often learned about these opportunities from other parents or searched them out independently. One mother suggested being given all relevant contact information to keep on file and being told about one or two key services they should contact early on. Ensuring caregivers were aware of services, grants, and subsidies they are entitled to and helping them apply seems clear-cut, but unfortunately appears to have been overlooked for a number of families we spoke to. It may also have been the case that information given soon after diagnosis was forgotten amidst overwhelming circumstances, or was not relevant to the family at the time; highlighting the importance of re-visiting these issues throughout the trajectory of a child's LLI. Members of the care team should be cautious of making assumptions about a family's financial status. Parents may feel uncomfortable acknowledging the issue with the health care team out of embarrassment and fear of being judged.

Posttraumatic Growth

The parent caregivers who participated in this study reported positive aspects of their situations. Quantitatively, they showed growth in all areas measured by the Posttraumatic Growth Inventory. Common themes that emerged from the parent interviews were consistent with the various aspects of growth—including experiencing new possibilities, enhanced relationships, enhanced strength, increased appreciation of life, and spiritual change (McMillen & Fisher, 1998; Tedeschi & Calhoun, 1995). Given the evidence that personal growth does occur in caregiving parents, social workers with an understanding of the aspects that comprise growth will be better situated to provide care to parents in pediatric palliative care settings. Their understanding of this construct will guide clinical interventions that could potentially enhance growth or assist families in exploring the associated changes.

Most research examining growth has concerned people who have experienced a traumatic occurrence that is of a single incident or shorter in duration (Aldwin et al., 1994; Burt & Katz, 1987; Dunn, 1994; Elder & Clipp, 1989; Silver, Boon, & Stones, 1983; Thompson, 1985). The presence of posttraumatic growth reported in the current study is significant because these parent caregivers continued to experience the stresses and strains of caring for their child with a LLI, as well as carrying on with living and possibly caring for other children. Parent caregivers experienced both ongoing stresses and growth simultaneously. This co-occurrence of negative and positive experiences was consistent with the models of Folkman (1997) and Tedeschi et al. (1998) that propose that distress continues despite the positive aspects individuals experience as they face adversity. It is important for social workers and other health care professionals to understand and keep in mind that growth involves ongoing stress. Positive changes do not eliminate, or even necessarily mitigate, the distress experienced by parents. Further research is required to fully understand this relationship and to better translate it into practice for all health professions.

Folkman's (1997) revised model of stress and coping includes meaning-based coping that can lead to positive emotions. Parent caregivers were sustained by the meaning they discovered, both in their child's diagnosis and through their caregiving experience. Much of the meaning made by parents was spiritual in nature. Spirituality, which is sometimes religious in nature, but often is not, is an important and undervalued resource in posttraumatic growth (Cadell, 2012). Spiritual change seemed to be a gateway for some parent caregivers, leading toward acceptance and further expressions growth, such as the identification of personal strengths and reaching out to support others.

Changes in how people relate to others is one of the central tenets of posttraumatic growth (McMillen & Fisher, 1998; Tedeschi & Calhoun, 1995). Valuing new and old relationships and striving to nurture personal connections are expressions of personal growth. Parent caregivers had a deep appreciation for the connections they made with people in similar circumstances, whether these meetings were face to face or over the Internet. One mother described the online community she was a part of as her "lifeline." Parents unacquainted with strategies for connecting to other caregivers and the advantages may be in doing so, will benefit from the guidance of a social worker who is knowledgeable and up-to-date on such opportunities, including information on local support groups, and contact information for national organizations and virtual networks and blogs. These resources can ease the sense of isolation for parents, ill children, and their healthy siblings. Supporting connections will benefit families living in rural communities, as well as those living in cities who have limited opportunities to leave the house to attend meetings due to their child's complex needs.

In what was possibly the most outward expressions of personal growth, caregivers were motivated by their own circumstances, or by what they saw happening around them, to take action. In becoming advocates, caregiving parents demonstrated personal strength and courage by sharing their stories or speaking out on issues that were meaningful to them. They worked on campaigns and organized community events to raise awareness of their child's condition and pediatric palliative care in general. Others addressed systemic issues by writing letters and petitioning government officials. Being empowered to work for a cause felt to be unjust or disregarded by the mainstream can have a ripple-effect on the positive changes experienced; both at a personal and societal level. In becoming advocates, parents who may have been consumed by their child's condition and caregiving role broadened their focus and applied their energy and passion in acts of altruism. Many of the caregivers in the current study commented that the reason they volunteered to participate was because they wanted to help others and influence how pediatric palliative care is provided. Advocating is possibly the most outward expression of growth that has implications for others, as well as the caregivers themselves. This is a little explored area of growth and merits further research attention. In addition, social workers may be able to assist in the facilitation of growth in parent caregivers by cultivating this altruism.

Caregiving parents shared their experiences of self-care rituals and routines that were associated with growth—including nurturing relationships, exploring new opportunities, and finding strength. Social workers should endeavor to have conversations with parent caregivers about their ability to cope, relationships at home and work, and strategies for caring for themselves on a regular and ongoing basis. A parent who might feel self-assured of his or her ability to manage one week, may feel completely overwhelmed the next. Health care providers could be of greater benefit to parents by critiquing their practices through a family-centered lens to evaluate what issues they may be avoiding and what services may be lacking. PPC is a complex field, with the physical health of the child being only one piece of a complex puzzle. Self-care as a mechanism for posttraumatic growth is worthy of further investigation.

LIMITATIONS

There are numerous limitations in this research. The most obvious is a self-selection bias which may influence both the quantitative and the qualitative data. The participants entered into the study knowing that both negative and positive aspects of the experience would be discussed. It is certainly possible that those who did not identify in any way with any positive aspect of their experience may not have agreed to participate. On the other hand, since so little is known about the positive aspects, particularly whether growth even occurs in this population, a self-selection bias is not necessarily a limitation; however, it is important that these results be interpreted as a sample of those who did want to answer questions about both the positive and negative aspects of a stressful experience, rather than being a representative sample of caregiving parents. Interview participants were also selected, in part, for geographic convenience; however, interviewers were located in several locations throughout Canada and the United States.

The quantitative sample is comprised of caregivers who were related to the ill child through a variety of relationships. The heterogeneity of the sample may be a limitation. The relatively small number of fathers, in relation to the mothers, may also have skewed the statistics. No special effort was made to recruit fathers other than asking each volunteer if there was anyone else in the family who might participate. It is important to specifically seek out fathers for pediatric palliative research as their experience is different (Davies et al., 2004) and underrepresented (Macdonald et al., 2010). The questionnaires were completed in the privacy of the participants' homes and, as such, we do not know who completed the survey although we have no reason to believe that participants would misrepresent themselves in this study.

Finally, with the qualitative data, the interviews that were conducted with couples may have resulted in some individuals not fully voicing their opinions, as a result of the relationship with the other person. However, those who were interviewed in pairs were invited to do so specifically as part of a project to discuss growth in couples, as this is an area where very little research has been done.

CONCLUSION

This research has provided many valuable lessons for social workers and other health care professionals working in pediatric palliative care. The parents' experiences of positive aspects and posttraumatic growth in the midst of the stresses of caring for their child with a life-limiting illness provide important insights to guide family-centered care. This is especially relevant for an emerging field of practice such as pediatric palliative care. When looking to improve a system one must go to the experts. Thus, only by inviting families to participate in research will we hear from the experts. And the message that parents want to participate in research was clearly demonstrated by the large number of parents who volunteered for this study, almost all of whom indicated they would like to be contacted about follow-up research.

The method of gathering both quantitative and qualitative data and allowing each to inform one another has provided a unique and important stage and audience for families to share personal stories and offer words of advice to palliative care professionals. The themes here of growth alongside distress, building connections, becoming an advocate, and growth through self-care are not all covered in the posttraumatic growth literature. These areas warrant further research.

Findings from the current study serve to inform social workers of the significance of these issues for parents and give voice to their perspective on such matters. As finances and growth of caregivers are considerations falling under the scope of practice of social work, it is hoped that this information will be utilized within the field to direct interventions that will ease distress and burden and enhance growth for families caring for a child with a life-limiting illness.

REFERENCES

Aldwin, C. M., Levenson, M. R., & Spiro, A., 3rd. (1994). Vulnerability and resilience to combat exposure: Can stress have lifelong effects? *Psychology and Aging, 9*(1), 34–44.

Ashby, M. A., Kosky, R. J., Laver, H. T., & Sims, E. B. (1991). An enquiry into death and dying at the Adelaide Children's Hospital: A useful model? *The Medical Journal of Australia, 154*(3), 165–170.

Association for Children with Life-Threatening or Terminal Conditions and their Families (ACT), Royal College of Paediatrics and Child Health (RCPHC). (2003). *A Guide to the development of children's palliative care services.* Bristol: UK.

Barakat, L. P., Alderfer, M. A., & Kazak, A. E. (2006) Posttraumatic growth in adolescent survivors of cancer and their mothers and fathers. *Journal Pediatric Psychology, 31*(4), 413–441.

Begun, A. (1993). Human behavior and the social environment: The vulnerability, risk, and resilience model. *Journal of Social Work Education, 29*(1), 26–35.

Benini, F., Spizzichino, M., Trapanotto, M., & Ferrante, A. (2008). Pediatric palliative care. *Italian Journal of Pediatrics, 34*(4). doi:10.1186/1824-7288-34-4

Bluebond-Langner, M., Belasco, J. B., Goldman, A., & Belasco, C. (2007). Understanding parents' approaches to care and treatment of children with cancer when standard therapy has failed. *Journal of Clinical Oncology: Official Journal of the American Society of Clinical Oncology, 25*(17), 2414–2419. doi:10.1200/JCO.2006.08.7759

Burt, M. A., & Katz, B. L. (1987). Dimensions of recovery from rape: Focus on growth outcomes. *Journal of Interpersonal Violence, 2*(1), 57–81.

Cadell, S. (2007). The sun always comes out after it rains: Understanding posttraumatic growth in HIV carers. *Health & Social Work, 32*(3), 169–176.

Cadell, S. (2012). Stress, coping, growth and spirituality in grief. In J. Groen, D. Coholic, & J. Graham (Eds.), *Spirituality in education and social work: An interdisciplinary dialogue.* Waterloo, ON, Canada: Wilfrid Laurier Press.

Cadell, S., & Sullivan, R. (2006). Posttraumatic growth and HIV bereavement: Where does it start and when does it end? *Traumatology, 12*(1), 45–59.

Cadell, S., Regehr, C., & Hemsworth, D. (2003). Factors contributing to post-traumatic growth: A proposed structural equation model. *American Journal of Orthopsychiatry, 73*(3), 279–287.

Calhoun, L. G., & Tedeschi, R. G. (1990). Positive aspects of critical life problems: Recollections of grief. *Omega, 20*(4), 265–272.

Contro, N., Larson, J., Scofield, S., Sourkes, B., & Cohen, H. (2002). Family perspectives on the quality of pediatric palliative care. *Archives of Pediatric & Adolescent Medicine, 56*(1), 14–19.

Corden, A., Sloper, P., & Sainsbury, R. (2002). Financial effects for families after the death of a disabled or chronically ill child: A neglected dimension of bereavement. *Child: Care, Health, & Development, 28*, 199–204.

Davies, B., & Howell, D. (1998). Special services for children. In D. Doyle, G. Hanks, & N. MacDonald (Eds.), *Oxford textbook of palliative medicine* (2nd ed., pp. 1077–1084). Oxford, United Kingdom: Oxford University Press.

Davies, B., Gudmundsdottir, M., Worden, B., Orloff, S., Sumner, L., & Brenner, P. (2004). "Living in the dragon's shadow": Fathers' experiences of a child's life-limiting illness. *Death Studies, 28*(2), 111–135.

Davies, B., Widger, K., Steele, R., Cadell, S., Siden, H., & Straatman, L. (2011). Research considerations in pediatric palliative care. In J. Wolfe, B. Sourkes, & P. Hinds (Eds.), *Textbook of interdisciplinary pediatric palliative care* (1st ed., pp. 96–103). Philadelphia, PA: Saunders.

Dunn, D. S. (1994). Positive meaning and illusions following disability: Reality negotiation, normative interpretation, and value change. *Journal of Social Behavior and Personality, 9*(5), 123–138.

Elder, G. H., & Clipp, E. C. (1989). Combat experience and emotional health: Impairment and resilience in later life. *Journal of Personality, 57*(2), 311–341.

Folkman, S. (1997). Positive psychological states and coping with severe stress. *Social Science & Medicine (1982), 45*(8), 1207–1221. doi:S0277953697000403 [pii]

Frantz, T. T., Trolley, B. C., & Farrell, M. M. (1998). Positive aspects of grief. *Pastoral Psychology, 47*(1), 3–17.

Gilmer, M. J., Foster, T. L., Bell, C. J., Mulder, J., & Carter, B. S. (2012). Parental perceptions of care of children at end of life. *American Journal of Hospice Palliative Medicine.* Advance online publication. doi:10.1177/1049909112440836

Goldman, A. (1996). Home care of the dying child. *Journal of Palliative Care, 12*(3), 16–19.

Ickovics, J. R., & Park, C. L. (1998). Paradigm shift: Why a focus on health is important. *Journal of Social Issues, 54*(2), 237–244.

Jones, B. (2005). Pediatric palliative and end-of-life care: The role of social work in pediatric oncology. *Journal of Social Work in End-of-Life & Palliative Care, 1*(4), 35–62.

Joseph, S., & Linley, P. A. (2008). *Trauma, recovery, and growth: Positive psychological perspectives on posttraumatic stress.* Hoboken, NJ: John Wiley.

Kessler, B. G. (1987). Bereavement and personal growth. *Journal of Humanistic Psychology, 27*(2), 228–247.

Kumar, S. P. (2011). Reporting of pediatric palliative care: A systematic review and quantitative analysis of research publications in palliative care journals. *Indian Journal of Palliative Care, 17*(3), 202–209.

Lazarus, R. S., & Folkman, S. (1984). *Stress, appraisal, and coping.* New York, NY: Springer.

Lehman, D. R., Davis, C. G., Delongis, A., Wortman, C. B., Bluck, S., Mandel, D. R., & Ellard, J. H. (1993). Positive and negative life changes following bereavement and their relations to adjustment. *Journal of Social and Clinical Psychology, 12*(1), 90–112.

Liben, S., Papadatou, D., & Wolfe, J. (2008). Paediatric palliative care: Challenges and emerging ideas. *Lancet, 371*, 852–864. doi:10.1016/S0140-6736(07)61203-3

Macdonald, M. E., Chilibeck, G., Affleck, W., & Cadell, S. (2010). Gender imbalance in pediatric palliative care research samples. *Palliative Medicine, 24*(4), 435–444.

Masten, A. S., Best, K. M., & Garmezy, N. (1990). Resilience and development: Contributions from the study of children who overcome adversity. *Development and Psychopathology, 2*, 425–444.

Masten, A. S., Best, K. M., & Garmezy, N. (1994). Resilience in individual development: Successful adaptation despite risk and adversity. In M. C. Wang & E. W. Gordon (Eds.), *Educational resilience in inner-city America: Challenges and prospects* (pp. 3–25). Hillsdale, NJ: Lawrence Erlbaum Associates.

McMillen, J. C. (1999). Better for it: How people benefit from adversity. *Social Work, 44*(5), 455–468.

McMillen, J. C., & Cook, C. L. (2003). The positive by-products of spinal cord injury and their correlates. *Rehabilitation Psychology, 48*(2), 77–85.

McMillen, J. C., & Fisher, R. (1998). The perceived benefit scales: Measuring perceived positive life changes after negative events. *Social Work Research, 22*, 173–187.

McMillen, C., Howard, M. O., Nower, L., & Chung, S. (2001). Positive by-products of the struggle with chemical dependency. *Journal of Substance Abuse Treatment, 20*(1), 69–79. doi:S0740547200001513 [pii]

Monterosso, L., Kristjanson, L. J., Aoun, S., & Phillips M. B. (2007). Supportive and palliative care needs of families of children with life-threatening illnesses in Western Australia: Evidence to guide the development of a palliative care service. *Palliative Medicine, 21*, 689–696.

Morrod, D. (2004). Make or break—Who cares for couples when their children are sick? *Sexual and Relationship Therapy, 19*, 247–263.

Park, C. L., Cohen, L. H., & Murch, R. L. (1996). Assessment and prediction of stress-related growth. *Journal of Personality, 64*(1), 71–105.

Parker, M. (1996). Families caring for chronically ill children with tuberous sclerosis complex. *Family and Community Health, 19*, 73–85.

Rapoport, A., Beaune, L., Weingarten, K., Rugg, M., & Newman, C. (2012). Living life to the fullest: Early integration of palliative care into the lives of children with chronic complex conditions. *Current Pediatric Reviews, 8*(2), 152–165.

Scannapieco, M., & Jackson S. (1996). Kinship care: The African American response to family preservation. *Social Work, 41*(2), 190–196.

Schneider, M., Steele, R., Cadell, S., & Hemsworth, D. (2011). Differences on psychosocial outcomes between male and female caregivers of children with life-limiting illnesses. *Journal of Pediatric Nursing, 26*(3), 186–199.

Silver, R. L., Boon, C., & Stones, M. H. (1983). Searching for meaning in misfortune: Making sense of incest. *Journal of Social Issues, 39*(2), 81–101.

Steele, R. G. (2000). Trajectory of certain death at an unknown time: Children with neurodegenerative life-threatening illnesses. *The Canadian Journal of Nursing Research (Revue Canadienne De Recherche En Sciences Infirmieres), 32*(3), 49–67.

Steele, R., & Davies, B. (2006). Impact on parents when a child has a progressive, life-threatening illness. *International Journal of Palliative Nursing, 12,* 576–585.

Tedeschi, R. G., & Calhoun, L. G. (1995). *Trauma and transformation: Growing in the aftermath of suffering.* Thousand Oaks, CA: Sage.

Tedeschi, R. G., & Calhoun, L. G. (1996). The Posttraumatic Growth Inventory: Measuring the positive legacy of trauma. *Journal of Traumatic Stress, 9*(3), 455–471.

Tedeschi, R. G., Park, C. L., & Calhoun, L. G. (1998). *Posttraumatic growth: Positive changes in the aftermath of crisis.* Mahwah, NJ: Lawrence Erlbaum Associates.

Thompson, S. C. (1985). Finding positive meaning in a stressful event and coping. *Basic and Applied Social Psychology, 6*(4), 279–295.

Thornton, A. A., & Perez, M. A. (2006), Posttraumatic growth in prostate cancer survivors and their partners. *Psycho-Oncology, 15,* 285–296.

Index

Note:
Page numbers in **bold** type refer to figures
Page numbers in *italic* type refer to tables